Welcome to ...

CLiC™

INTERNATIONAL

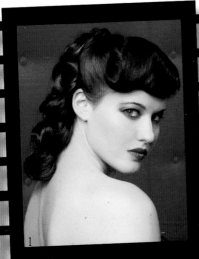

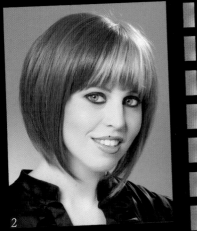

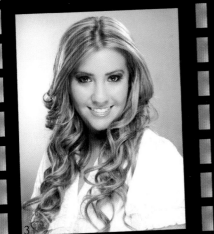

CLiC™ INTERNATIONAL

CERTIFIED LEARNING IN COSMETOLOGY™

The Spectrum of Light™

haircoloring

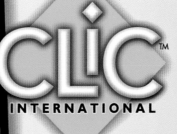

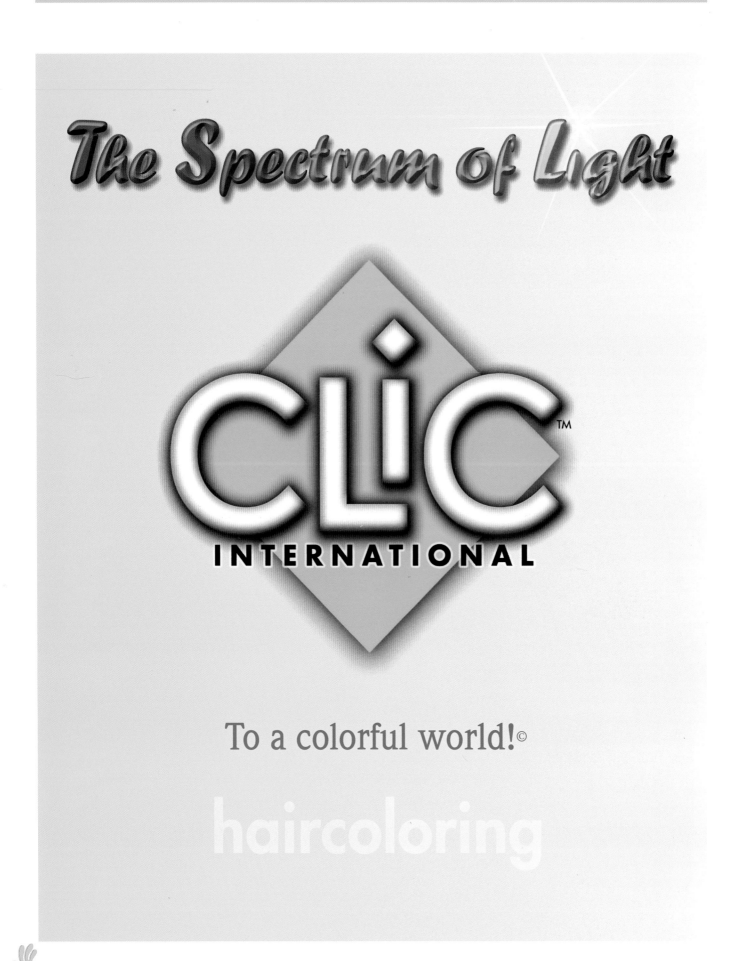

The Spectrum of Light

CLiC
INTERNATIONAL

To a colorful world!©

haircoloring

Dedication ...

This haircoloring module is dedicated to the scientists, artists, professionals and manufacturers of the past and present who have given us the visual illumination of haircolor.

"Thank you for your hard work and dedication. You have given us a colorful world!"

CLiC ART DEPARTMENT:

Layout, Design and Illustration

Senior Graphic Artist
Rae L. Baker

Graphic Artists
Artemus D. Tuisl
Janelle C. Klitsch

Research Technical Writer
Lorrie C. Weinhold

SPECIAL ACKNOWLEDGEMENTS

Photographer
Mickey Donatelli
Randy Donatelli
Shelly McGinnis

Editor
Lori McFerran

Index
Potomac Indexing, LLC
www.potomacindexing.com

Subject Matter Experts
Carol A. Massaro
Claudia S. Carothers
Jonathan Schonning
Karen Tenpas
Lindsey Watts
Marc Galgay
Marge Binner
Margie L. Wagner-Clews
Paul Sites
Robin J. Sebastian
Sylvia Boulware
Theresa Andrews
Theresa Ksyniak
Timothy Jarmillo
Yvette Caballero

Proofreading
Diane M. Grustas
Lorraine Letcavage

CLiC Photo Shoot Contributors
Beth Ann Miller for Goldwell
Judith Deardorff for Goldwell
Marge Binner for Goldwell
Randy Rick
Sherry Winters for Goldwell

Haircolorists
Beth Ann Miller for Goldwell
Judith Deardorff for Goldwell
Marge Binner for Goldwell
Sherry Winters for Goldwell
Robert Willis International/
Fingerblades Inc.

"A special thanks to all the professionals who shared their artwork, products and scientific information to educate and inspire future cosmetologists. Your photographs demonstrate the variety of effects that can be achieved through creativity and dedication!"

HAIRCOLORING/ page(picture number)

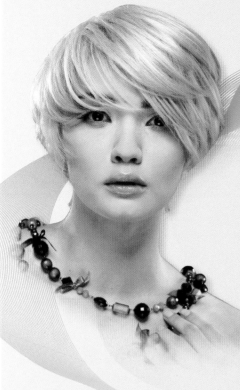

Hairdesign Contributors:

Bob Steele Salon
steelehair@bobsteelehair.com
1(1), 81(1), 182(1), 287(2), 289(1)

Carmen Carmen Salon
183(1)

Currie Hair, Skin and Nails
117(1), 127)1), 135(1)

Daniel Pereyra–
Vogue Hair Design
287(3)

Dina Culotta –
Ladies & Gentlemen Salon
289(3)

DJ Moran/Grund Hair
20(1), 289(4), 293(2)

Duncan Lai
123(8)

Frederick's Salon & Spa
121(1)

Honey -
Robert Willis International
123(1)

Jenniffer & Co. Salon & Spa
73(3), 79(3), 84(2), 123(7,9),
288(2), 291(2)

Jessica Jurker –
Brown Aveda Salon
287(1)

Josh Carpenter-Costner–
Carmen Carmen Salon é Spa
8(1)

Kara Landiak –
Tangles Salon
290(1)

Kate Wohek & Megan Harford –
Casal's de Spa & Salon
154(1)

Ladies and Gentlemen Salon & Spa
72(1), 288(1)

Lauren Houser –
Kathy Adams Salon
290(2)

Lauren McDonald –
Kathy Adams Salon
128(1)

Leslie Cook –
Tangles Salon
73(1), 129(2)

Oak Street Hair Group
154(2)

Pat's Hair Design & Color Group
1(2), 79(2), 110, 123(4), 129(1), 228(3)

Philip Bataglia –
Focus Salon
182(2)

Randy Rick
291(1)

Rob Willis International/
Fingerblades
21(1), 107(2), 123(1,3), 158(3),
228(1), 294(1)

Robin Cook –
Tangles Salon
14

Michelle Anderson-Savvy
Salon & Spa
51(1)

Tammy Hylton –
Above and Beyond Salon & Spa
18(1)

The Brown Aveda Institute
17(1), 22(1), 73(4), 135(2), 258(1)

The Ohio Academy Paul
Mitchell Partner School
102, 293(1)

Yellow Strawberry Global Salon
1(3), 9(1), 51(2), 73(2), 123(6), 158(2)

Makeup Contributors:

Ashley Brown –
Savvy Salon & Spa
51(1)

Betty Mekonnen –
Tangles Salon
73(1), 129(2), 290(1)

Gina Payne -
Sheer Professionals Salon
182(2)

Natalie Stapleton –
Carmen Carmen Salon é Spa
8(1)

Rachel Jacobsen –
Kathy Adams Salon
290(2)

Tia Makosky –
Casal's de Spa & Salon
154(1)

Foreword ...

Sir Isaac Newton once said, "If I have been able to see further, it was only because I stood on the shoulders of giants." This profound statement represents one of the guiding principles of the Certified Learning in Cosmetology® (CLiC) system. There is much to be learned and discovered by "standing on the shoulders of giants." It is only by studying the discoveries and accomplishments of leaders who came before us that we can prepare for the future.

The CLiC system provides a broad cosmetology education with a focus on three key areas:
1- A basic cosmetology foundation
2- An introduction to artistic concepts and visual inspiration to nurture creativity
3- Effective interpersonal, sales and retail techniques

Although the professional cosmetology industry is continually evolving, the fundamentals remain unchanged.
The basis of cosmetology is an understanding of human biology combined with scientific and mathematical theories used to create desired results. Building on the basic concepts of cosmetology, we explore artistic and visual inspiration in order to develop and nurture creativity. Throughout the foundational and artistic learning process, successful interpersonal sales and retail skills are introduced and practiced. These skills are paramount to the personal satisfaction and financial success of the professional cosmetologist.

CLiC is a visually stimulating and inspirational system, focused on preparing students to be salon-ready upon completion of their studies.
Master hairdesigner and international award winner Randy Rick is the creative force behind the revolutionary CLiC system. Always a step ahead, Mr. Rick developed the CLiC system of learning to elevate the artistic, practical and marketable skills of today's students. Through the CLiC program, he shares his vast international knowledge and experience with you ... the professional cosmetologist of the future!

CLiC to a colorful world!

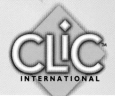

Introduction to CLiC ..

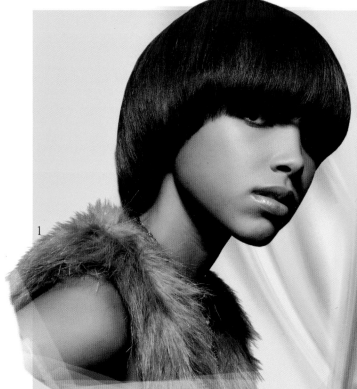

1

You are about to begin an exciting journey into the world of cosmetology. The Certified Learning in Cosmetology® (CLiC) system will be your road map, leading you to realize the rewards of becoming a successful, professional cosmetologist.

The CLiC system is designed to enhance fundamental cosmetology education by incorporating artistic inspiration and successful salon service and retail skills. The learning modules cannot possibly cover all cosmetology art fashions, but will always encourage freedom of expression and innovation to adapt to future trends.

This revolutionary system focuses on meeting your educational needs with a solid, competency-based cosmetology curriculum. Each CLiC module is designed to develop manual dexterity, professional perception, tactile sensitivity and the artistic vision used in the industry. Each module will take you through our competency-based learning system, which will progress from simple to complex skill levels, utilizing the methods of practice, experimentation and testing.

The CLiC educational system is presented in individual learning modules, each consisting of a complete program. The module system enables you to focus on individual disciplines, by offering courses for certified specialization in each field. This ensures the opportunity to learn and develop the skills needed for a rewarding and profitable career in the cosmetology field of your choice.

For additional information, contact:

CLiC INTERNATIONAL®
396 Pottsville/Saint Clair Highway
Pottsville, PA 17901 USA
1.800.207.5400 USA & Canada
001.570.429.4216 International
1.570.429.4252 Fax

www.clicusa.com

Introduction to Haircoloring ...

Light from the sun illuminates our world in a brilliant spectrum of colors. People learned to create and develop these colors into various art forms. There are elements of art in everything we see, touch and feel in our lives.

Studying historical art from the masters helps inspire the development of future trends in fashion. Haircoloring is just one artistic medium in the broad world of cosmetology and fashion.

THE ARTISTRY ...

Every artist, regardless of the medium in which he or she works, must begin by learning the necessary tools and techniques specific to his or her chosen art. Studying the work of artistic masters is also an important part of the learning process. Learning about haircoloring is much the same.

THE CHEMISTRY ...

The journey to achieve superior artistry in haircoloring takes continual study and experimentation. You must understand the physical properties of the spectrum, as well as the chemical products used to create haircolor.

It is a highly technical and sophisticated field of study, but mastering the scientific principles of haircoloring will yield the ability to create extraordinary works of haircolor art.

THE INSPIRATION ...

Mastering any art form requires learning simple, intermediate and complex skills. This book will provide many visual examples to inspire your creativity and facilitate the learning process.

Continuing Education ...

If you are the type of person who desires to be the "best" and takes an "above and beyond" approach in your technical and practical skills ...
then become a Mastercolorist!!!

What is a Mastercolorist?

A professional stylist who pursues a higher degree of education and develops expert practical skills in the art of haircoloring – other terms used to recognize this type of achievement are Haircolor Expert, Color Specialist or Certified Haircolorist.

A variety of haircolor manufacturers offer their own advanced haircoloring courses under continuing education to achieve this career status. You can also connect with the American Board of Certified Hair Colorist at www.haircolorist.com to research their program. In addition, some states offer Mastercolorist certification as part of their continuing education for the stylist.

Most continuing education programs consist of a written test along with an examination of step-by-step advance color procedures. Comprehensive materials and face-to-face training seminars will effectively assist you in preparing and practicing for the evaluation.

Benefits of becoming a Mastercolorist:

- Achieve specialized industry status and greater career potential
- Expand your haircoloring skills and creativity
- Greater income/earning power
- Increase your confidence and image
- Encourage and inspire other professionals toward future career development

Introduction to Icons ...

"Hello! My name is CLiCer, and I am your personal tour guide to the many fields of cosmetology. In this book, we will be studying the art of Haircoloring. I will lead and encourage you as we explore the many facets of haircoloring tools and techniques. I will give you tips, ideas and reminders for each of the topics to assist you during the learning process. Welcome! I am excited to have you join me for this journey of learning."

Regulatory Alert

Whenever you see the **Regulatory Alert** icon, it will remind you and your instructor to check governmental regulations about the subject on the page. The rules and regulations for cosmetology vary according to geographic location. Place a sticker, from the back of the book, over the shadow if there are governmental regulations that must be followed in your area.

The 3Rs

At the conclusion of your services there are three important steps you should consistently follow. **Retail** professional products to your customers for home maintenance. **Re-book** future appointments to encourage regular visits. Ask for **referrals** to broaden your customer base. By following the 3Rs they will improve your income and profitability as a professional cosmetologist.

CLiCer's Sales Pointers

As you will learn throughout this book, selling and financial skills will be just as important to your success in the salon as your actual knowledge and skills in the field of cosmetology services. Whenever you see this icon with CLiCer's hand, pay special attention to the **sales pointers** you are given. Combining sales skills with cosmetology art skills will create a dynamic force for your salon success!

Interactive Tags

Microsoft Tags, or QR Codes, are essentially readable web links. Users can download the free reader application for internet-capable mobile devices with cameras. The user takes a photo of the tag and is instantly directed to electronic information available in a variety of formats – such as text, videos, photos, and more. Use the Tag Codes in the book to explore gateways to interactive media and internet data.

Table of Contents ...

Table of Contents ...

Inspiration . . .

Nature's beautiful
array of colors
can be your
inspirational guide.

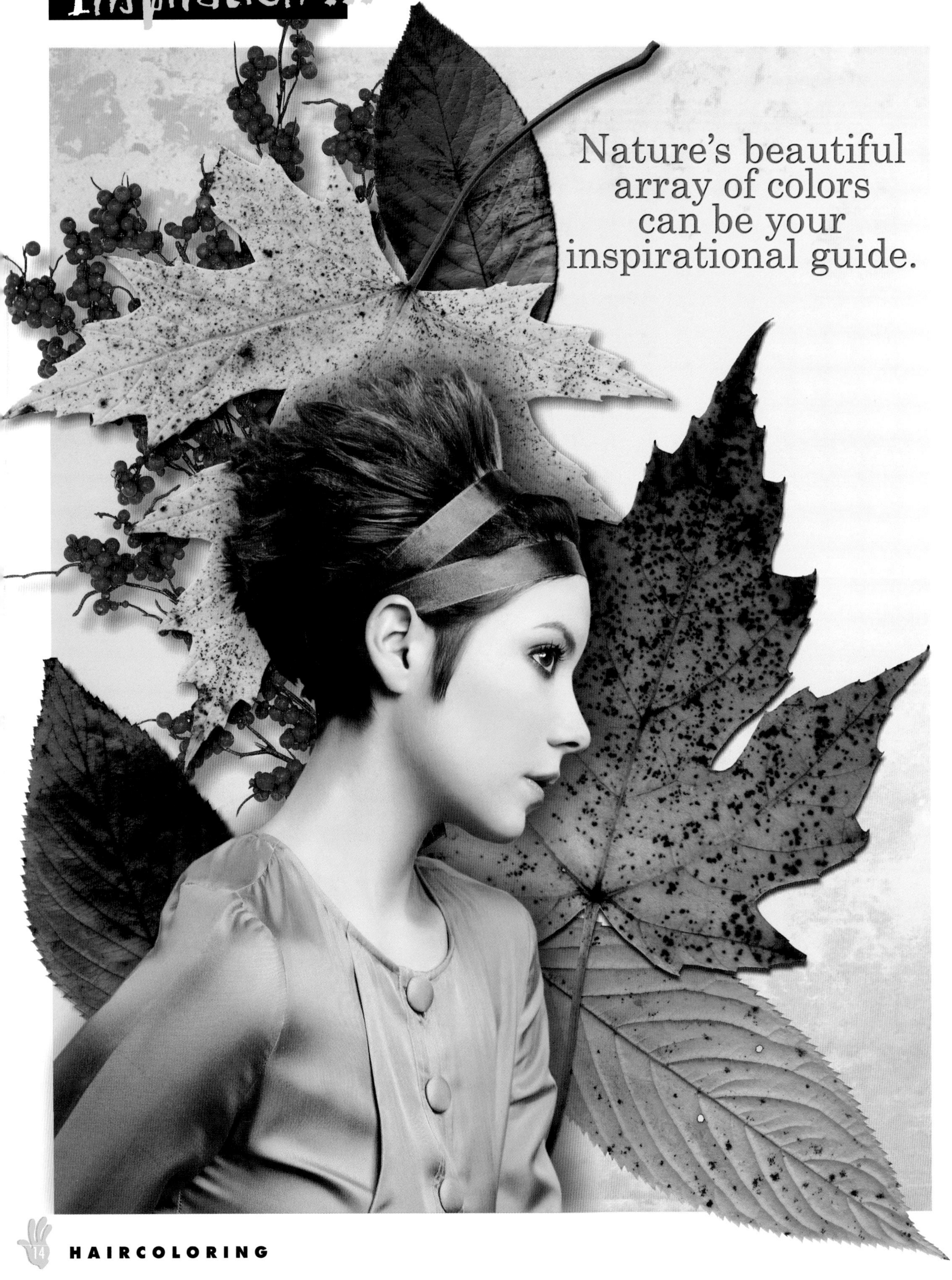

formula hue

metallic oxidation

pigments

porosity

viscosity

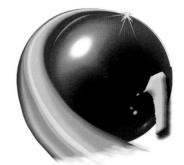

Terminology

Terminology ...

Haircoloring vocabulary is the language of the professional haircolorist. As artists master these words, it will give them a competitive edge as professional haircolorists when marketing haircolor services to existing and future client/guests.

Allergy is when the body reacts with a hypersensitive response to a normally harmless substance.

Atom is the smallest part of an element consisting of neutrons, protons and electrons.

Color is a physical phenomenon of light or visual perception associated with the various wavelengths seen by the eye.

1

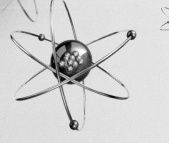

THE COLOR WHEEL

Color Wheel is used as a visual support for the law of color to show how all 12 colors are created.

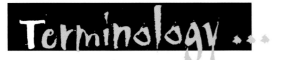

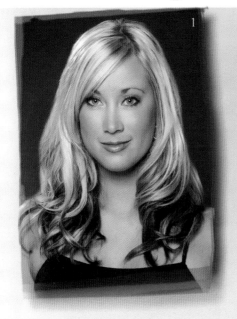

Decolorizing, also referred to as **decapping,** is the action of lightener scattering or breaking up the natural or artificial pigments in the cortex of the hair.

Deposit occurs when color molecules enter the cuticle and/or cortex layers of the hair.

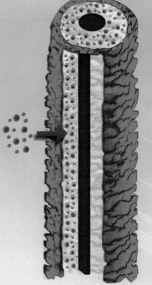

Developer is an oxidizing agent also known as hydrogen peroxide and is added to haircolor or lightener to assist in the development process.

Double Process is a procedure that includes two separate procedures: first step is to pre-lighten (decolorize) hair and second step is to deposit (recolorize) haircolor.

1 DECOLORIZE

2 RECOLORIZE

Terminology...

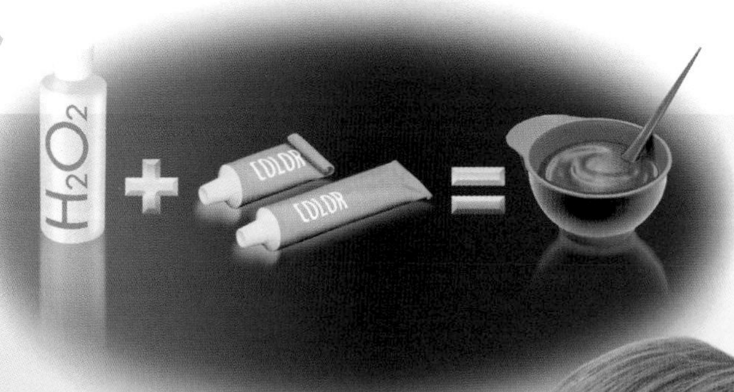

Formula is a mixture of haircolor products used to create the desired shade – the "recipe" used by the haircolorist to color the client/guest's hair.

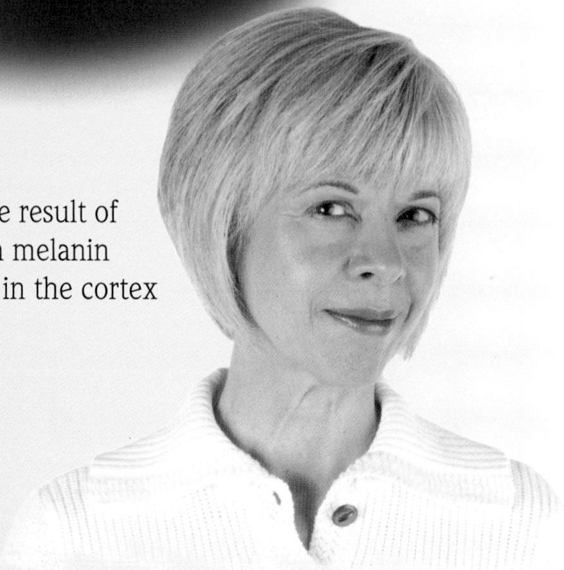

$$H_2O_2 + COLOR\ COLOR = $$

Gray Hair is the result of a gradual decline in melanin production located in the cortex layer of the hair.

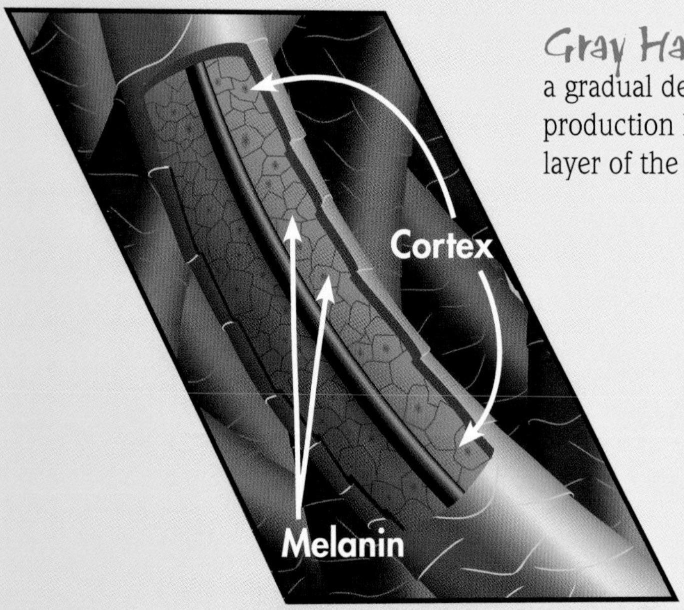

Cortex

Melanin

Haircolor is the melanin located in the cortex layer and/or the artificial pigments from actual haircoloring products that are responsible for providing color to the hair.

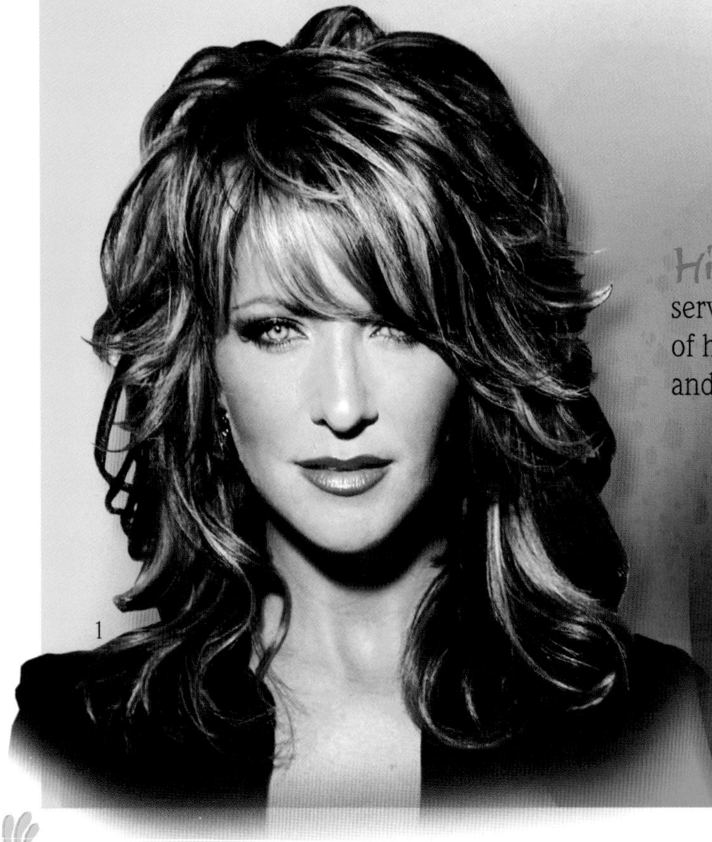

Highlighting is a special effects service that lightens selected pieces of hair with the use of lightener and/or haircolor.

1

Hue is the general name for color.

Hydrometer is an instrument that measures the specific gravity of a liquid (an example is hydrogen peroxide).

Hydrometer

Level is determining the degree of lightness to darkness of a color depending on how much light is reflected or absorbed.

Lightening is when haircolor or lightener is applied, causing the natural or artificial pigments in the hair to lift to higher levels of color. It is the opposite of going darker.

Line of Demarcation is a dark band (or visible line) that is a result of haircolor overlapping onto previously colored hair.

Before New Color

After New Color

Line of Demarcation

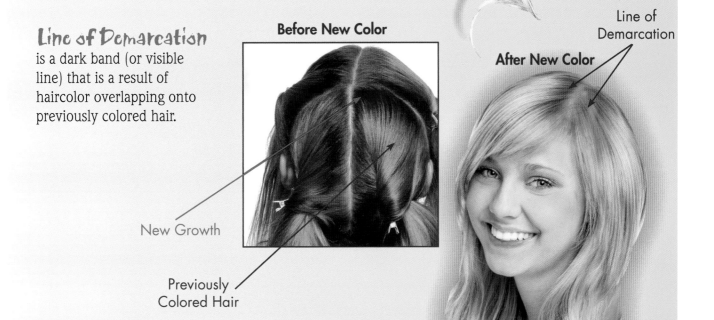

New Growth

Previously Colored Hair

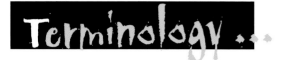

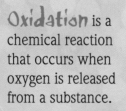

Lowlighting is a special effects service that deposits medium to dark shades of haircolor on selected pieces of hair, thereby creating dimension to the hairdesign.

Melanin is the coloring matter that provides us with the natural color of our hair and skin.

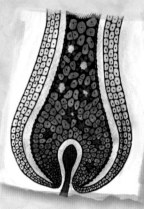

1

Metallic Materials are various types of metals used in non-professional haircoloring products that create a slow progression of color to the hair.

IRON

Silver

COPPER

Oxidation is a chemical reaction that occurs when oxygen is released from a substance.

O²

Overlapping is when color or lightener is applied and spreads onto previously colored hair creating a visible line of demarcation or a dark band.

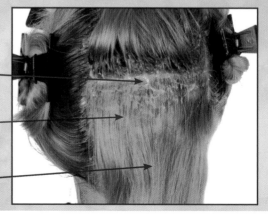

Regrowth with New Color

Overlap of New Color on Previously Colored Hair

Previously Colored Hair

Terminology ...

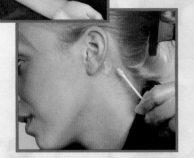

Patch or Predisposition Test
is applying a small amount of haircolor mixture on the skin to check for skin sensitivity of product/chemical.

pH Scale
is the measurement of hydrogen ion concentration in a solution to determine if it is acid, neutral or alkaline.

10,000,000	**0**	Acid
1,000,000	**1**	
100,000	**2**	
10,000	**3**	
1,000	**4**	
100	**5**	Average pH of hair
10	**6**	
1	**7**	NEUTRAL "pure" water
10	**8**	
100	**9**	
1,000	**10**	
10,000	**11**	
100,000	**12**	
1,000,000	**13**	
10,000,000	**14**	Alkaline

Pigments
are what give color its color, whether the source is natural, chemical or mineral.

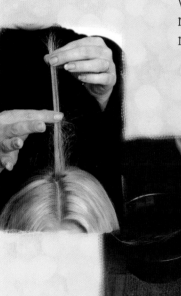

Porosity
is the amount of water/liquid the hair (cuticle) absorbs within a relative amount of time.

Saturation
is a combination of pigment concentration and light reflection, which results in a multitude of colors.

PERMANENT

1

Terminology ...

Strand Test is performed before or during a haircolor service by placing color or lightener on a small subsection of hair; process, rinse and dry hair for client/guest and professional to preview the end color result or during processing to determine if color is properly developed.

Toner is a light level (pastel or pale) of haircolor used on pre-lightened hair, which may range from semi-permanent to permanent haircolor.

Red undertone

Undertone is the underlying or base color seen within the predominant color. It can be a result of the natural inborn pigments, or artificially created to produce a two-level effect.

1

White Hair has a total absence of pigment – no melanin in the cortex layer.

Viscosity is the property of a fluid or semi-liquid in which the flow is resisted; the thickness or heaviness of the liquid.

Inspirational Quotes ...

"If you care enough for a result, you will most certainly attain it."

William James, professor of psychology, Harvard University, 1875

"We can do more than dream of being great — we can practice, practice and practice until those dreams become real."

- Randy Rick, Founder of CLiC International

"Whoever does not love his work cannot hope that it will please others."
- Unknown

"In a constantly changing world, one dares not stand still or become complacent or repetitive."

Renato Brunas, CLiC Haircoloring Book contributing editor

"THE GREATER THE DIFFICULTY ... THE GREATER IS THE GLORY."
- **Cicero**, ancient Roman philosopher

"A promise is a commitment."

- Unknown

"The best confidence builder is experience!"

Unknown

"'Imagination' is the art of seeing the unknown."

Randy Rick, Founder of CLiC International

"Better to ask twice than to go wrong once."

- German proverb

"Determine never to be idle ...it is wonderful how much may be done if we are always doing."

Thomas Jefferson, third President of the United States

Haircoloring Terminology REVIEW QUESTIONS

FILL-IN-THE-BLANKS

A.	Allergy
B.	Atom
C.	Color Wheel
D.	Decolorizing
E.	Deposit
F.	Double Process
G.	Formula
H.	Gray Hair
I.	Highlighting
J.	Hue
K.	Hydrometer
L.	Level
M.	Metallic Materials
N.	Oxidation
O.	Pigments
P.	Porosity
Q.	Predisposition Test
R.	Undertone
R.	Viscosity
T.	White Hair

1. _____ is the result of a gradual decline in melanin production in the cortex layer of the hair.

2. _____ give color its color.

3. _____ is the property of a fluid in which the flow is resisted – the thickness or heaviness of the liquid.

4. _____ is determining the degree of lightness to darkness of a color depending on how much light is reflected or absorbed.

5. _____ has a total absence of pigment – no melanin.

6. _____ is the smallest part of an element.

7. _____ is a special effects service that lightens selected pieces of hair.

8. _____ is used as a visual support for the law of color to show how all 12 colors are created.

9. _____ is the absorption of water/liquid into the hair (cuticle) within a relative amount of time.

10. _____ is the procedure that includes two separate procedures: first step is to pre-lighten and second step is to deposit haircolor.

11. _____ is a chemical reaction that occurs when oxygen is released from a substance.

12. _____ occurs when the color molecules enter the cuticle/cortex layers of the hair.

13. _____ is an instrument that measures the specific gravity of liquid.

14. _____ is the underlying or base color seen within the predominant color.

15. _____ is applying a small amount of haircolor mixture on the skin to check for skin sensitivity.

16. _____ is the general term used for color.

17. _____ is a hypersensitive response to a normally harmless substance.

18. _____ are various types of metals used in non-professional haircoloring products.

19. _____ is the action of lightener diffusing the natural or artificial pigments in the cortex of the hair.

20. _____ is a mixture of the haircolor products used to create the desired shade.

STUDENT'S NAME   DATE   GRADE

developer   foils

henna   filler

timer   hydrometer

toner

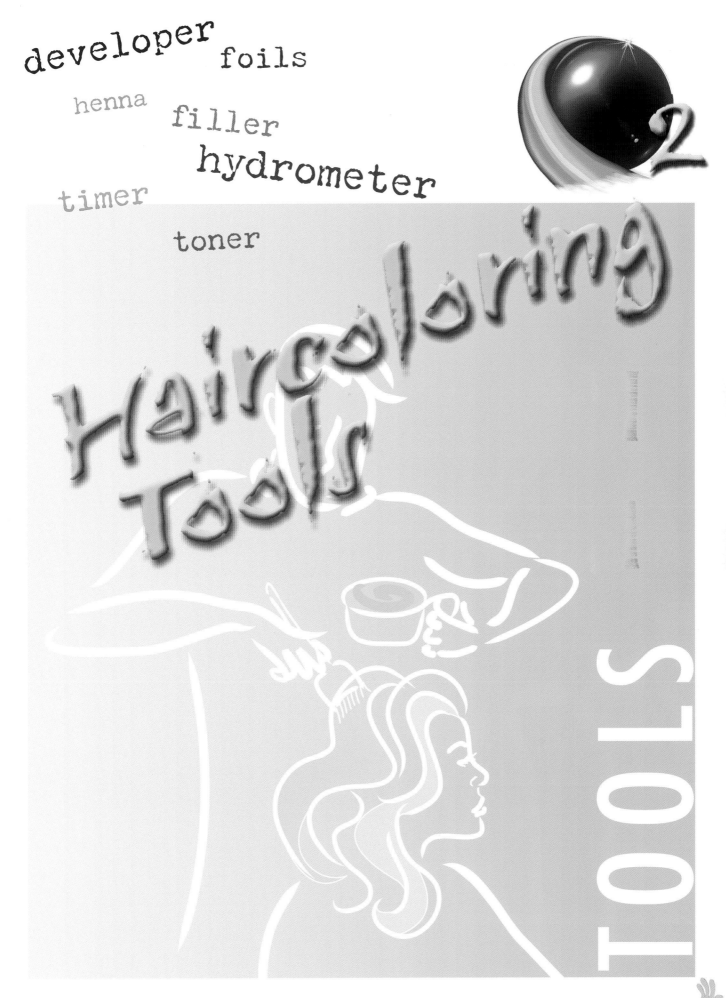

Haircoloring Tools

TOOLS

Haircoloring Tools Introduction ...

Whether you *are a carpenter, bank teller, teacher or cosmetologist,* **the proper tools are essential to ensuring a job well done.** *It is important to learn how to apply these tools in a safe and effective manner in order to ensure a successful end result.*

As a professional haircolorist, the proper tools used will benefit both you and the customer/guest. Purchasing and using the appropriate tools will build self-assurance for formulating, measuring, mixing and placement of color, which then **creates accuracy and accuracy delivers success – AND success ensures a happy, loyal customer/guest.**

1

Haircoloring Tools Introduction ..

1

Some **manufacturers produce their own tools*** to be used in conjunction with their haircolor products. To obtain optimal results, we recommend that you purchase the **necessary tools to accommodate the particular haircolor product** you are using. If for any reason a question or problem should arise during the service, most manufacturers have a hotline number or website to refer to for troubleshooting.

2

CAUTION: Never combine different color lines due to the numerous chemical arrangements that take place within each formulation of color. A manufacturer will usually create a "product friendly" line that is compatible with its product collection.

*Keep in mind while a number of professional tools are covered in this chapter, there may be other tools available, as the marketplace is constantly expanding and innovative techniques and tools are being introduced.

Safety and Protection Tools...

To professionally and successfully color a client/ guest's hair, various types of chemical products are formulated and mixed together. If not properly handled some of these haircoloring products may **produce skin irritation and/ or stain and damage a client/guest's as well as the artist's clothing.** For this reason as professionals, we must take the responsibility to **ensure the safety and protection of our client/guests as well as ourselves.**

Chemical Apron or Smock is made of a high quality, stain-resistant vinyl or cloth material that can be **worn by the professional** as an outer layer. It will help **protect your clothing** from chemical damage and stains.

Gloves are manufactured from latex, vinyl and synthetic materials to **protect hands from stains and chemical sensitivity** and to **ensure client/guest safety.**

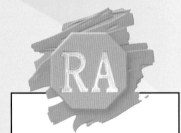

RA

Gloves are required to be worn for all cosmetology services in many localities.

CAUTION: Some people have allergies or sensitivities to latex. Be sure to ask your client/ guests prior to wearing latex gloves before haircoloring service.

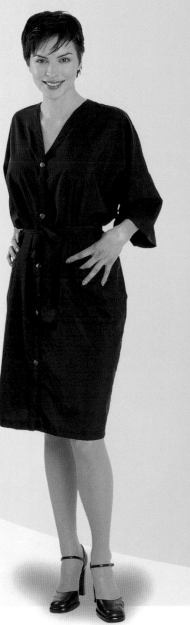

Robes are worn by the customer/guest during a haircolor service to **eliminate possible chemical staining or seepage** onto client/guest's clothing. Client/guests receiving haircoloring services are recommended to change into a robe prior to service. Robes are made of a washable material that provides **comfort and easy access** along the neck and hairline for color application.

"The salon/spa should provide the necessary protective clothing and/or accessories for its client/guests as well as for the professionals."

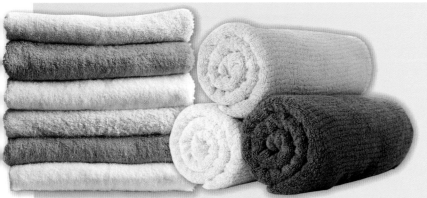

Safety and Protection Tools ...

Cloth Towels are made from an absorbent washable material and create a protective barrier by **preventing skin-to-cape and/or skin-to-skin contact** with service tools or liquid products. Towels are also used to remove moisture from hair and dry hands after shampooing.

Disposable Towels made from non-woven fabric provide a lint-free surface on which to **place tools** during haircolor service. These towels **eliminate the need for laundering** and are used as an alternative to the cloth towel for draping the client/guest.

Magnet Closure

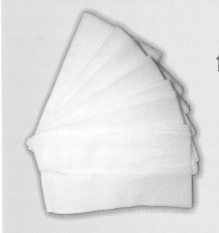

Capes are used to **cover client/guests' clothing to protect from damage** during all hair services. Capes are available in different materials, lengths, widths and colors, and have a variety of closures including Velcro®, hooks, ties, magnets and snaps. Most capes are machine washable, but not all are dryer safe. Read manufacturer's instructions prior to use.

Elastic Collar

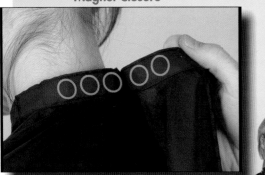

Safety and Protection Tools ...

Neck Strips are wrapped around the client/guest's neck to **prevent skin-to-cape contact.** They also help to **catch water or chemical liquids** that may possibly escape during a service. Neck strips are available in paper or cloth and come in different widths and lengths.

Draping for Chemical Services (haircoloring)

Neck strip

Towel

Cape

Towel

RA

Please check with local regulatory agency for the required chemical draping in your area.

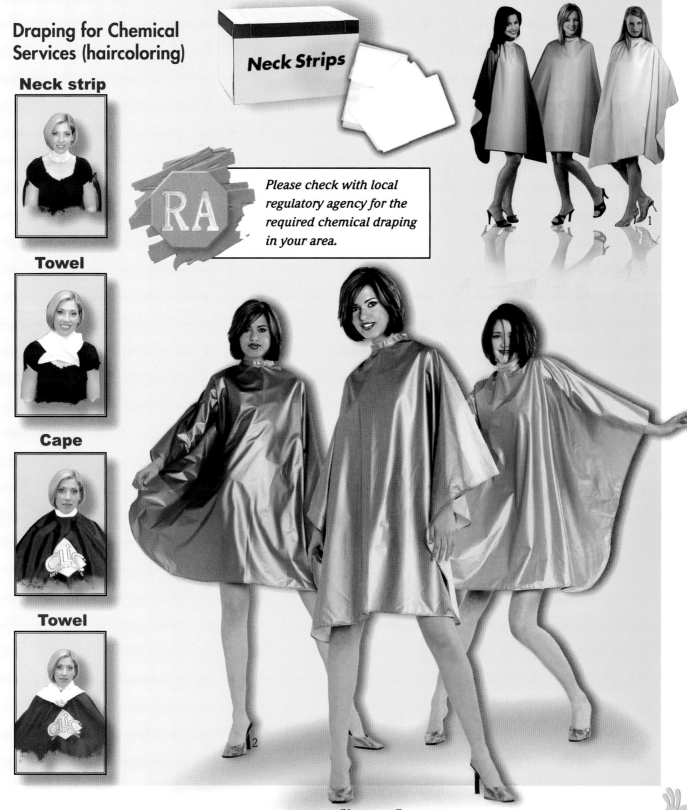

Protective Cream is a cosmetic cream or lotion applied along the client/guest's hairline prior to haircolor application. The cream **protects the skin** from possible sensitivity, irritation and color staining.

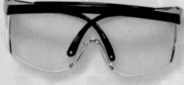

1

Safety Glasses are lightweight eye wear that provide **eye protection** upon the handling of haircolor products and during the service. These glasses keep the eyes **safe from accidental splashing** that may occur when mixing chemical products.

RA

Many regulatory agencies require that safety glasses be worn for certain haircoloring services.

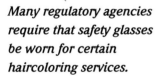

Cotton is used to **apply color for a patch test** and may be **placed around hairline** to prevent the color from dripping. Depending on color technique, small strips of cotton are **placed between subsections along the base or scalp area** to avoid color from seeping or overlapping onto previously colored hair.

Safety and Protection Tools ...

Dust Masks are disposable and worn by the professional to help **protect the respiratory system as a result of inhaling powdered chemicals** while mixing a haircolor formula.

CAUTION: The mask will not adequately protect from vapor or fume inhalation.

Air Purification (pu-ri-fi-ca-tion) **System** is available to **clean the air** within the salon. The technology in some of today's air filtration systems is so advanced that the systems actually **eliminate chemical odors** caused by mixing haircolor chemicals. In addition, the air is cleansed of bacteria, fungi and virus particles that inevitably enter the salons.

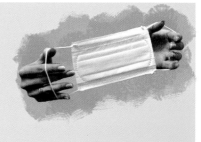

1

Wet Disinfection (dis-in-fec-tion) **System** is a sanitizer used for implements that are exposed to client/guests' skin and nails. Tools are **completely immersed** in jars or special containers filled with a disinfectant solution for the allotted time determined by following manufacturer's directions. Implements must be **cleaned before immersion** by removing all hair and using a cleaning solution of soap and water.

2

BARBICIDE
DISINFECT
FUNGICIDE &

Dry Disinfection (dis-in-fec-tion) **System** is a sanitizer that employs an ultraviolet light in a cabinet. Tools are **placed inside after being cleansed and disinfected** with a commercial solution. This keeps the disinfected combs and brushes sanitary until needed for next service.

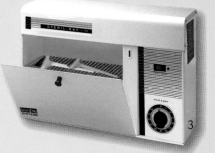

3

Color Bowl and Brush Usage ...

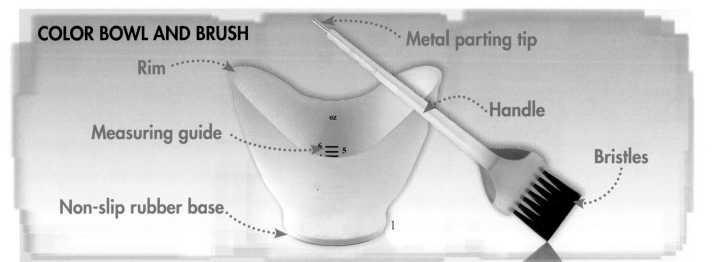

COLOR BOWL AND BRUSH

Metal parting tip

Rim

Handle

Measuring guide

Bristles

oz
6 ≡ 5

Non-slip rubber base

1

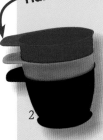

Handle

2

Haircoloring (hair-col-or-ing) *Bowls* are used to **hold color or lightener mixture.** These bowls vary in features; some have **measurement guides** on the inside, or they may feature an **edge along the bowl's rim** in which to rest the color brush. Most bowls will have a **non-slip rubber base** to prevent the bowl from moving and some **contain a scale** that weighs the color formula. Bowls are available in various sizes and colors and come in plastic or glass.

Haircoloring Brushes are commonly referred to as tint brushes, which perform **neat and accurate applications of color or lightener on the hair.** The handle supplies stability while the color or lightener is placed on the hair with the bristles. Brushes are available in assorted sizes, lengths and designs. The design of the brush is chosen according to the type of haircoloring service performed.

3

Placement: The nylon bristles of the brush hold the color or lightener mixture until placed directly on the hair. Grasp the handle of the brush and scoop the desired amount of color according to hair texture and type of color application.

Control: Grasp the handle of the brush in-between thumb, index and middle fingers. The amount of pressure applied when placing the brush's bristles against the hair will force the color onto the subsection of hair. In this way, thorough coverage is accomplished, which enables the hair to absorb the color or lightener.

Key Elements:

✔ The tip of the brush handle may be used to create partings and subsections during the color or lightener application

✔ Special effects are created when using color brushes with various bristle designs

✔ Colors or lighteners with a thick consistency are best suited for a bowl and brush color application

Metal parting tip of brush handle

Color Bowl and Brush Dynamics ...

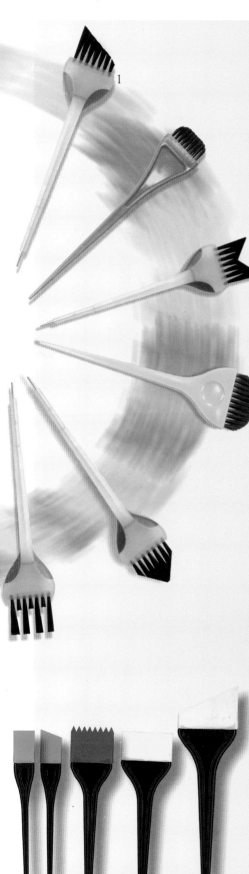

Dynamics for Using a Bowl and Brush

1 Grasp handle of color brush in-between thumb, index and middle fingers.

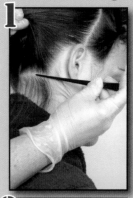

2 Use plastic or metal tip of brush handle to part a ¼ inch (0.6 cm) subsection of hair.

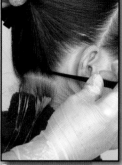

3 Place bristles of brush into color mixture.

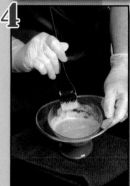

4 Pull brush from color mixture –showing amount of mixture on the bristles at end of brush.

5 Swipe opposite side of brush on edge of bowl to remove excess color mixture from bristles.

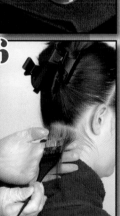

6 Hold subsection of hair with opposite hand and place bristles onto subsection of hair.

7 Continue to place color along subsection of hair.

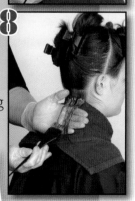

8 Cover subsection of hair according to color procedure being performed.

NOTE: Steps 6 thru 8 color application depends on type of color procedure.

Applicator Bottle Usage ...

APPLICATOR BOTTLE

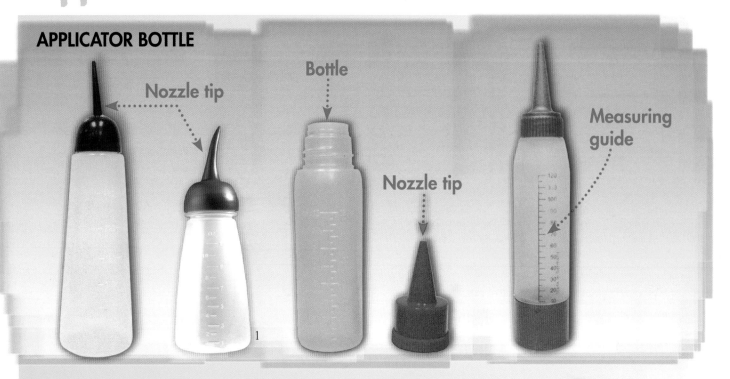

Nozzle tip

Bottle

Nozzle tip

Measuring guide

Applicator (ap-pli-ca-tor) **Bottles** are used to **hold the color or lightener mixture** and **apply liquid or low viscosity types of color or lightener.** The bottle is plastic with a nozzle tip applicator from which the haircolor is dispensed. Some nozzle tip designs are used in place of the comb to part the hair into subsections. Bottles are marked to include ounce (oz.) or metric (ml) measurements and come in an assortment of sizes and designs.

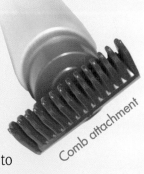

Comb attachment

Placement: Hold the bottle with your dominant hand in an upright position until ready to apply color or lightener. Slowly turn the bottle to enable the color product to flow out from nozzle tip in a controlled manner.

Control: The amount of pressure used to squeeze the color product from the bottle will determine the flow of color dispensed. A strong pressure squeeze will force more product onto the hair, whereas a light pressure squeeze will place a smaller amount of product on the hair.

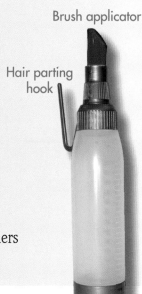

Brush applicator

Hair parting hook

Key Elements:

✔ The nozzle tip may be used to create partings and subsections during the color or lightener application

✔ Faster and easier color application

✔ Great safety and control of low viscosity (thickness) type colors or lighteners

Applicator Bottle Dynamics ...

DYNAMICS FOR USING AN APPLICATOR BOTTLE

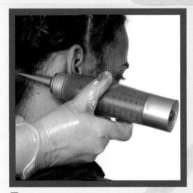

1. Grasp applicator bottle in same manner as pencil or pen.

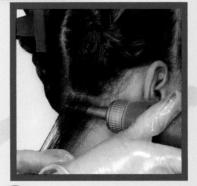

2. Use nozzle tip to part a ¼ inch (0.6 cm) subsection of hair.

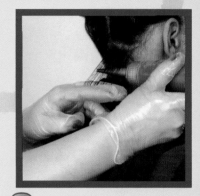

3. Hold subsection of hair with opposite hand.

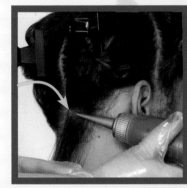

4. Place nozzle tip at scalp along parting.

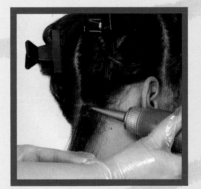

5. Squeeze out the amount of color needed for accurate coverage.

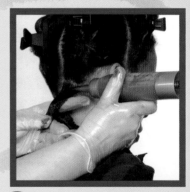

6. Use nozzle tip to spread color along subsection of hair.

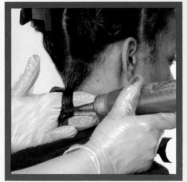

7. Continue to place color onto subsection of hair.

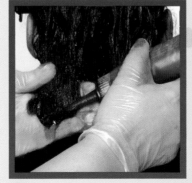

8. Cover entire subsection to the hair ends.

NOTE: Steps 6 to 8 color application is only when color is applied scalp to hair ends.

Hydrometer Usage ...

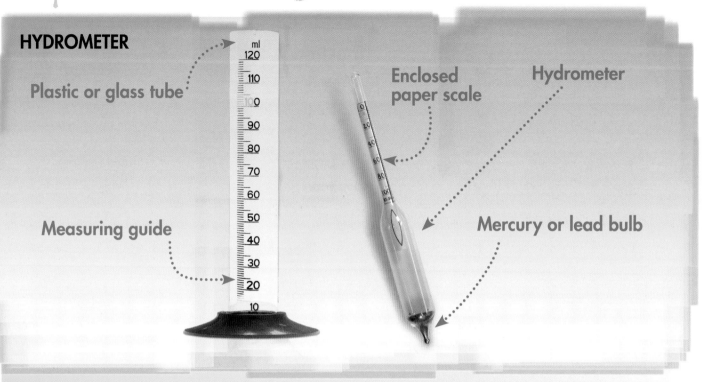

HYDROMETER

Plastic or glass tube

Enclosed paper scale

Hydrometer

Measuring guide

Mercury or lead bulb

Hydrometer (hy-drom-e-ter) is an instrument that **measures the specific gravity of a liquid** – in this case, the liquid is hydrogen peroxide. It generally appears as a long, thin, glass stem with a mercury or lead-filled bulb at one end. A paper scale is enclosed in the stem to determine the reading of the liquid's specific gravity. The hydrometer will **float depending on the number of times the liquid is lighter or heavier than water.** For hydrogen peroxide the hydrometer will determine the volumes of oxygen gas available, therefore revealing the true strength.

Placement: A clear (liquid) hydrogen peroxide is poured into the glass or plastic tube. The lead-filled bulb or hydrometer is placed into the liquid.

Control: Plastic or glass tube is placed on flat surface and held by fingers and thumb of dominant hand. Liquid hydrogen peroxide is poured by opposite hand. The hydrometer will float in the liquid gauging an approximate strength.

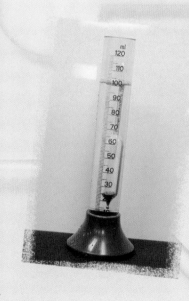

Key Elements:

✔ Confirms accuracy of hydrogen peroxide strength, whether using a brand new bottle or a used bottle

✔ Quick and easy measuring tool

✔ Can create different volumes of hydrogen peroxide if needed

Hydrometer Dynamics ...

NOTE: A cream developer **cannot** be measured for specific gravity or strength due to viscosity (thickness) of product.

Objectives for testing hydrogen peroxide strength:

- Checking the strength of a new bottle of hydrogen peroxide

- Checking the strength of a half-empty bottle of hydrogen peroxide

- Create two different volumes of liquid hydrogen peroxide from a single source using distilled water

Hydrometer Dynamics for Testing the Strength of Hydrogen Peroxide

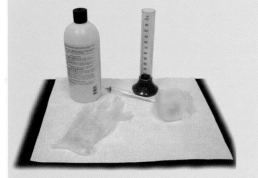

1. Set out materials of hydrogen peroxide, hydrometer, gloves, disposable towel and measuring cup.

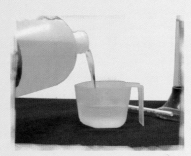

2. Place measuring cup on flat surface and pour 3 to 4 ounces of hydrogen peroxide into cup.

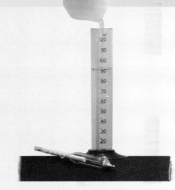

3. Pour hydrogen peroxide into tube.

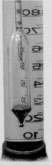

4. Place the glass hydrometer into the plastic tube.

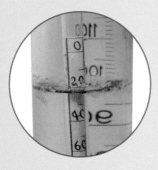

5. Allow the hydrometer to float to the measurement line indicating the exact strength of hydrogen peroxide.

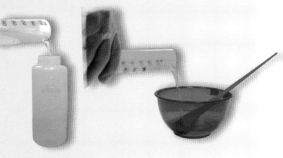

6. Dispose of or pour hydrogen peroxide into color bowl for mixing. Sanitize/clean hydrometer and measuring cup.

Haircoloring Tools ...

When applying professional haircolor, there are particular tools needed to **perform a safe and effective service.** Sometimes manufacturers recommend special types of tools be purchased **for accurate formulation of color and safe placement of color.** The following is an overview of some haircoloring tools that professionals use to formulate, measure, mix and apply haircolor.

Tube Wringer (wring-er) is an easy-to-use tool that lets you **squeeze every bit of color from its tube.** Place and secure the wringer at the end of color tube; turn the dial counter-clockwise till you get to the ounce mark on the tube or squeeze out entire contents of tube. This is a great money saver for the salon!

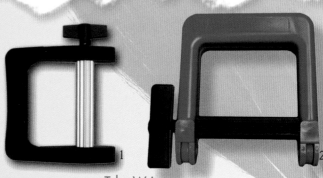

Tube Wringer

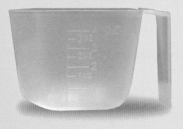

Measuring Cup is marked **indicating units of measurement** in milliliters (ml), ounces (oz.) or cubic centimeters (cc). This measuring device will provide an **accurate amount of product needed** for each color formula.

NOTE: Some color product manufacturers create their own measuring tool that is compatible with their color line.

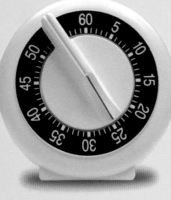

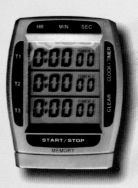

Timers are pre-set devices that will automatically stop at the set time for a coloring service, which indicates the **processing time is complete.** This will remind the colorist to either strand test and/or remove the client/guest's color.

Salon Imaging System is a computer program that allows the **professional to input an image of the client/ guest,** and then change the picture to show him or her different hairstyles, haircolors and makeup. **Client/guests are able to view themselves with various changes** and see the style, haircolor and makeup that best complements them.

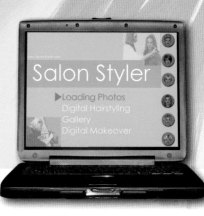

Haircoloring Tools ..

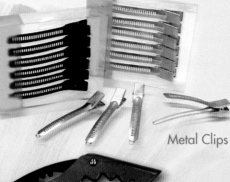

1

Metal Clips

2 Plastic Clip

3

Plastic Clips

Hair Clips are used to **hold hair in a sectioned area** of the head. The clips control the hair and allow the **haircolorist to be neat and orderly** when applying color. Clips come in various designs, colors and sizes depending on length and texture of hair. Plastic clips are recommended for use in all chemical services.

Color Swatch Chart is a catalog of **hair, which visually displays the colors** from a manufacturer's product line. This is a great asset for the professional haircolorist and can be used as a guide to determine the client/guest's natural and desired color, as well as viewing the family of colors and their intensifiers.

4

Color Key is inserted at end of the color tube to remove color. Turn the key **to dispense the color** following the number guide alongside tube as reference for the accurate amount needed. This tool is smaller, but performs in the same fashion as the tube wringer.

Color Mixer

Color Key

Color Key

Color Mixer is a tool that will **automatically mix the color or lightening mixture.** This enclosed device with beater-type attachments eliminates the need for the professional to mix and provide a smooth, creamy consistency.

5

Top View
Color Mixer

CAUTION: Avoid excessive beating of color mixture. This may increase the oxidation process.

Color Mixer

Tools for Special Effects ...

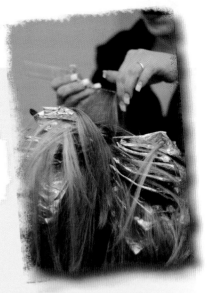

Creating special effects in haircolor gives you the **opportunity to use your imaginative and artistic ability.** There are many different tools available to inspire your creative thoughts and to apply your techniques. Some of the special effect tools provide a faster delivery, while others will assist in the technique and the creation of the color.

Pop-up Foil is a device that **separates each foil** therefore allowing the professional to obtain foil faster and easier. As each foil is removed, the next foil will cling to the adhesive strip located under the handle or arm ready for next pick. ▶

1

Thermal Wraps are an alternative to using foil. This **thermal wrap retains heat**, which assists in processing. Only one fold is needed to secure the hair/ color and the wrap is removed easily from the head without pulling or tugging on the hair. ▶

wrap

Hi-Lite Wraps
Hi-Lite Wraps
Hi-Lite Wraps
Hi-Lite Wraps

3

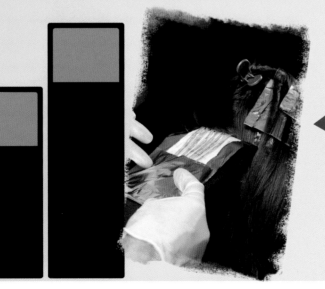

◀ **Foil Board** is a **supportive device** on which to **rest the foil** to accomplish a smooth and accurate placement of color or lightener. It offers control of the foil and hair when placing color or lightener onto the hair. This tool is especially helpful when foiling long hair.

2

Coloring Combs are used to section and subsection hair for color application as well as **achieve the weaving and slicing techniques used with foil placement.** These combs provide ease and accuracy to any haircoloring service. They are manufactured in a variety of designs and sizes, allowing the professional to select what will work best artistically and ergonomically.

NOTE: Always check with the color manufacturer before combing color through hair.

Traditional Color Comb or Shampoo Comb is a **wide-tooth comb used to distribute haircolor evenly** from scalp to hair ends. This comb is great for removing tangles before or after the service.

Streaking (streek-ing) **Comb** is used to help **create subtle or heavy bands of color** in the hair. The penetration of the comb's teeth will determine the amount of color applied. The **highlighting comb** performs much the same as the streaking comb, creating multiple textures – highlights, bands or ribbons of color.

STREAKING COMB

Three-in-One Comb is a comb, pick and brush combination, which is a versatile tool for the professional. This one comb **can do it all when applying the color** – eliminating the need for additional haircolor combs and brushes.

HAIRCOLOR CAP AND HOOK

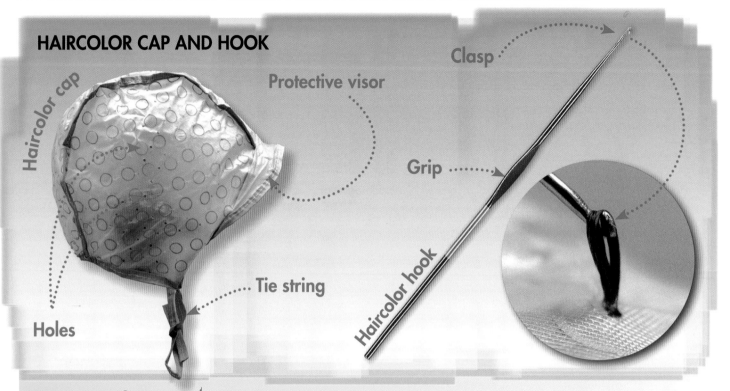

Haircolor cap

Protective visor

Clasp

Grip

Holes

Tie string

Haircolor hook

Haircolor or Lightener (light-en-er) **Cap** is designed for frosting, tipping, highlighting and lowlighting. It is manufactured in plastic, synthetic or latex materials with some caps having the option to be exposed of directly after use. The **cap consists of holes through which a pre-determined amount of hair is pulled.** Depending on end result, hair can be pulled from every hole or every other hole. A **haircolor hook** is used to **pull the hair through the holes.** The hook is made of plastic or metal and consists of a bulb-type clasp at one end, which grasps the hair under the cap and pulls the hair out of the hole.

Placement: The cap is positioned over the head starting at the forehead and pulled down to the nape area. It should have a snug, but comfortable fit.

Control: Hold the color hook in-between thumb, index and middle fingers and place at opening of hole. Insert hook at a forty-five degree angle through the hole to grasp amount of hair desired ... gently push hook through hole to avoid injury to the scalp. To create uniformity, obtain hair only from perimeter of the hole – do not push the hook further under the cap.

Key Elements:

✓ Ideal for special effects on short to medium length hair

✓ Creates a faster application of color or lightener on selected strands of hair

✓ Provides a safe application for lightener to not come in contact with skin or scalp

Haircolor Cap Dynamics

1.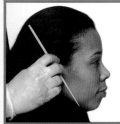
Comb hair back or comb the hair following the hair-design pattern.

2.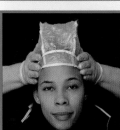
Position front of cap at forehead.

3.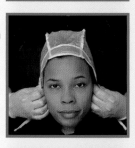
Pull cap back to cover entire head down to nape area.

4.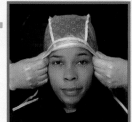
Pull cap down over sides of head resting either directly above the ears or covering the ears.

5.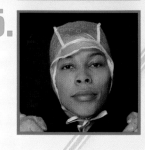
Optional: Some color caps are fastened with a tie string under the chin to hold cap in place and create a snug fit.

NOTE: Some color caps require powder to be placed on the inside or a plastic processing cap is used to cover the hair before the color cap is positioned on the head. This allows the color cap to glide easily over the head; it creates a smoother fit and helps to eliminate product leakage.

Haircolor Hook Dynamics

1.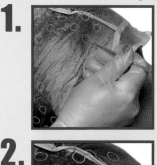
Holding the hook in-between thumb, index and middle fingers, place the clasp at opening of hole.

2.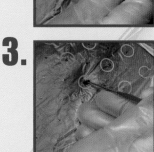
Insert the clasp at a forty-five degree angle into opening – piercing through the plastic.

3.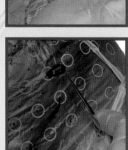
Loop hair through the clasp – the amount of hair taken depends upon the final result.

4.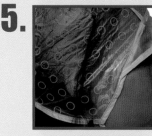
Pull clasp out of hole along with the hair.

5.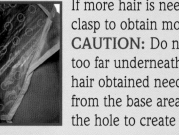
If more hair is needed, re-insert clasp to obtain more hair. **CAUTION:** Do not stick the hook too far underneath color cap. The hair obtained needs to be directly from the base area surrounding the hole to create uniformity.

6.
Continue pulling hair from other holes until desired amount is obtained. The hairdesign will determine the amount of hair being pulled.

Haircoloring Foil Usage ...

HAIRCOLOR FOIL

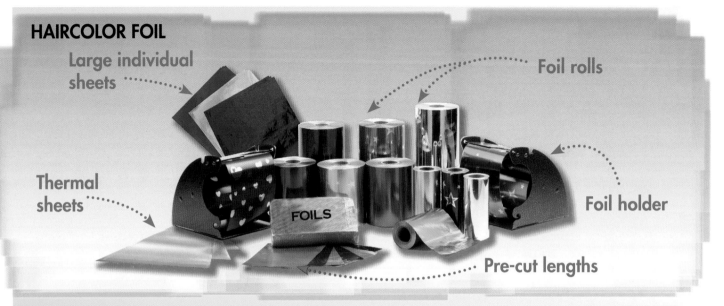

Large individual sheets

Foil rolls

Thermal sheets

FOILS

Foil holder

Pre-cut lengths

Professional Haircoloring Foil is used to **isolate subsections of hair being colored or lightened from the remaining hair that is not receiving color.** Foil is available in assorted colors, lengths and designs in order to match all haircoloring and highlighting services. The packaging for the foil varies depending on manufacturer, but typically comes in pre-cut lengths, rolls or individual full sheets, which are then cut at a certain length to accommodate the hair length and color application.

Placement: The foil rests against the scalp with a selected amount of hair (weaved or sliced) situated on top of the foil. Haircolor or lightener is applied on the selected strands of hair, which are placed on foil.

Control: A fold is created at one end of the foil using the tail of the comb. The folded end of the foil is situated at the scalp underneath the subsection of hair and held in place by thumb and index finger of opposite hand. Once color or lightener is applied, foil is folded in half to enclose the hair and to keep foil in place.

Key Elements:

✓ Ideal for creating dimensional haircoloring techniques

✓ Can be used for any length hair; best results on medium and long length hair

✓ Great versatility in color designing due to hair selection — some hair is colored or highlighted and some hair is not

Foil Dynamics

1. 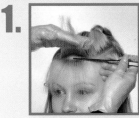 Subsection a pre-determined amount of hair.

2. 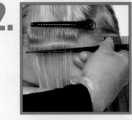 Perform a weave or sliced dimensional hair technique.

3. 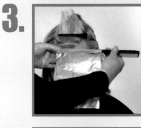 Using an adequate length of foil (determined by hair length), insert tail of comb under the fold (lip) of foil.

4. 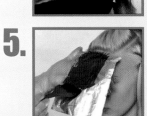 Place foil underneath subsection of hair, slide comb out of fold with opposite hand holding hair and foil in place.

5. 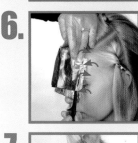 Apply color or lightener product to full length of hair subsection – fold foil in half.

6. 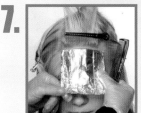 Fold both sides of foil to secure hair inside packet.

7. **Completed foil packet.**
CAUTION: Be careful not to press directly down onto foil in order to prevent the color or lightener from squeezing out on the hair and creating a line of demarcation.

Alternate Method

1. 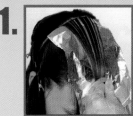 Place a subsection of hair on the foil.

2. 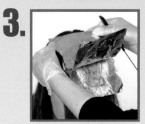 Place lightener or color product onto the hair.

3. 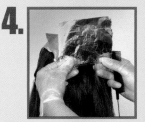 Place another piece of foil on top of hair, covering hair and product.

4. 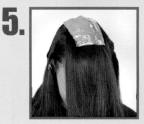 Fold the two pieces of foil in half to secure packet.

5. Fold both sides of foil inward to secure hair inside packet.

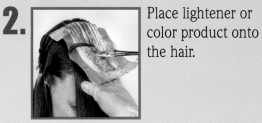

Liquid Haircoloring Tools ...

Liquid haircoloring tools are all the **liquid components necessary to color the hair.** There are a multitude of color manufacturers that produce a wide variety of color products in numerous forms. Generally, **color is classified in four categories** depending on the penetrating ability of the artificial pigments into the hair shaft. The four main types of color are **temporary, semi-permanent, demi-permanent and permanent.**

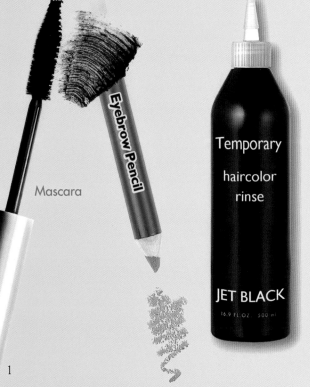

Mascara

Eyebrow Pencil

Temporary haircolor rinse

JET BLACK
16.9 FL.OZ.   500 ml

1

Temporary (tem-po-rar-y) **haircolor coats the surface/cuticle layer** of the hair shaft. Typically this type of color will **wash out of hair at next shampoo** depending on cuticle condition and consistency of color applied. This type of color will **only add or deposit color** to the client/guest's existing natural or artificial haircolor. The color directly in the bottle will be the color that goes on the hair – no mixing with other chemicals is required. Temporary color is manufactured in many forms, whether it is a shampoo, rinse, mousse, crayon, gel, pencil or spray-on color. Mascara and eyebrow color are also considered forms of temporary color.

Semi-permanent (se-mi-per-ma-nent) **haircolor penetrates the cuticle layer** of the hair shaft. This type of color will **gradually fade** depending on how often hair is shampooed and the condition of the cuticle **... may last four to six shampoos.** However, if hair has a severe porosity (raised cuticle scales), more absorption or deposit of color will ensue, but more fading may also occur due to poor cuticle condition. There is no mixing with another product – color in bottle is the color placed on the hair, and therefore this is a **deposit-only color.**

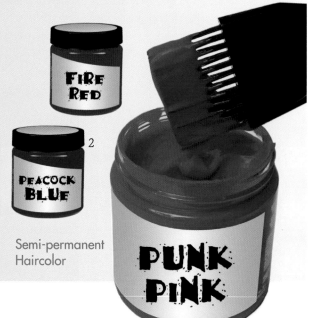

FIRE RED

PEACOCK BLUE

2

Semi-permanent Haircolor

PUNK PINK

Liquid Haircoloring Tools...

Demi-permanent (de-mi-per-ma-nent) **haircolor** **penetrates the cuticle and partially into the cortex layers** of the hair shaft. This type of color is **mixed with a low volume hydrogen peroxide**, which allows for further penetration into the hair shaft. Demi-color will **only deposit or add color to the client/guest's existing color,** and does not lighten the hair. Generally this type of color fades in **four to six weeks** depending on how often hair is shampooed and condition of cuticle.

Permanent (per-ma-nent) **haircolor penetrates into the cuticle and cortex layers** of the hair shaft. This type of color can **deposit and lighten the natural pigments** located in the cortex layer. Permanent color is **mixed with various strengths of hydrogen peroxide,** which enables the color to penetrate into the cortical layer. **It lasts until new hair growth appears** and a retouch of color is required.

DEMI-PERMANENT

PERMANENT

"Detailed information on each type of haircolor will follow in Chapters 4 and 5!"

Auburn

Permanent Haircolor

Golden Blonde

Permanent Haircolor

7G

hazel

7RG

cayenne

Permanent Haircolor

Liquid Haircoloring Tools ...

Lightening Powder

Lighteners (light-en-ers) **will lift/lighten the hair permanently by diffusing, dissolving or decolorizing the natural or artificial pigment in the cortical layer** of the hair shaft. The lightener is **mixed with various strengths of hydrogen peroxide** to create the oxidation needed for penetration into the cortex. It comes in **oil, cream or powder forms** and depends on the color service, product manufacturer and hair condition to decide which form is used.

Lightener

200 g ℮ net wt

Lightener

Toner is a **light level (pastel or pale) of haircolor** used on pre-lightened hair, which may range from semi-permanent to permanent. Toners are placed on pre-lightened hair to **deposit the required color tone and/or neutralize an undesirable color.** If using a demi-permanent or permanent color, hydrogen peroxide is added to formula mixture.

Toner

Liquid Haircoloring Tools ...

Color Filler is a product that **adds a missing primary color, deposits color on faded hair and/or equalizes the porosity of the cuticle layer** therefore creating uniform color results. Fillers are used prior to the application of a permanent color and usually come in a semi-permanent or demi-permanent form with high concentrations of pigment. There is also **conditioner fillers**, which even out porosity by placing conditioning agents into the cuticle layer to ensure even color absorption. Conditioner fillers can be applied as a separate service or prior to a haircolor application.

Concentrates (con-cen-trates), **Drabbers** (drab-bers), **and Intensifiers** (in-ten-si-fi-ers) are products that **contain undiluted pigments that are mixed into an existing color formula.** These colors can improve vibrancy, neutralize any undesirable color tones or be used alone on pre-lightened hair to create fun, bold and exciting color results.

Haircolor Remover is a manufactured product that reverses the oxidation of the artificial pigments in the cortex layer of the hair. This product is used if the haircolor results produced unwanted tones or the haircolor became too dark. The haircolor remover is applied directly after the haircoloring service to produce optimal results, but always check the manufacturer's directions.

Color Stain Remover is a product that **removes color staining on the skin** along the hairline and ears. Apply remover to a small amount of cotton and wipe over the skin where the staining occurred.

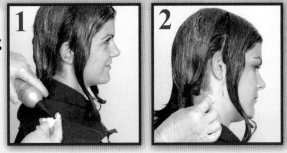

NOTE: For further detailed explanation of hydrogen peroxide volumes, refer to Chapter 5.

10 VOLUME OR *3%

20 VOLUME OR *6%

30 VOLUME OR *9%

40 VOLUME OR *12%

*EUROPEAN STRENGTH

Hydrogen Peroxide,

(hy-dro-gen per-ox-ide) referred to as **developer or catalyst** (cat-a-lyst), is an **oxidizing agent that is mixed with haircolor and lightener** prior to application on the hair. Hydrogen peroxide is essential in the development of demi-permanent, permanent and lightening formulas.

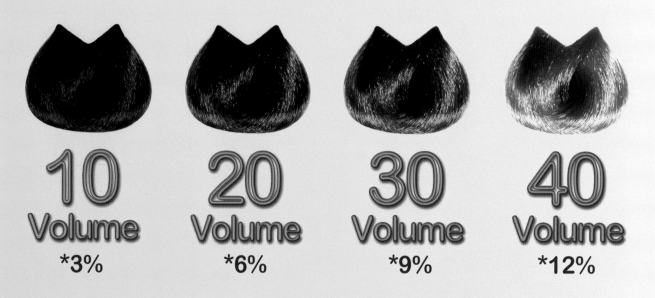

10 Volume *3%   **20 Volume** *6%   **30 Volume** *9%   **40 Volume** *12%

Developer is manufactured in **various strengths, referred to as volumes or percentages,** which means the amount or percentage of oxygen gas that is released from the product. **Commonly used volumes or percentages by the cosmetologist in the salon are 10, 20, 30 and 40 ... with 20 volumes as the overall choice.** Hydrogen peroxide also comes in three consistencies or forms; liquid, cream and dry. The selection of both the volume and the form of hydrogen peroxide is dependent upon the color manufacturer's instructions, type and kind of haircolor, and the service technique performed.

Liquid Haircoloring Tools ...

The consistencies of hydrogen peroxide are liquid, cream and dry.

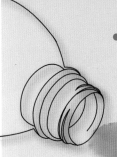

- **Liquid Hydrogen Peroxide** is the easiest and most versatile form of peroxide. Liquid developer is the ONLY form of peroxide that can be tested for its volume strength using the hydrometer.

Liquid Hydrogen Peroxide

> **CAUTION:** Liquid peroxide is clear and resembles water ... keep in a safe, cool and dry area and away from children and anyone not educated in the field of cosmetology. Apply this caution to all forms of hydrogen peroxide.

- **Cream Hydrogen Peroxide** performs the same as liquid developer, but contains thickeners, conditioners and in some cases even colors. The added thickeners help to prevent liquid color mixtures from dripping or running down the skin. Cream peroxide can be mixed with liquid or cream haircolors.

CREAM PEROXIDE

Cream Hydrogen Peroxide

Dry Hydrogen Peroxide

- **Dry Hydrogen Peroxide** comes packaged in powder, crystal or tablet form. This form of peroxide is not as common, but may be added to the liquid hydrogen peroxide to increase its strength and/or haircolor or lightener formulations for added processing boost.

Henna (hen-na) **Haircoloring**
is a **pure, natural product producing a
brown to red-orange color** in the hair.
Henna (hen-na), or *Lawsonia inermis* (Latin),
is a small tree or bush native to Turkey,
the Middle East and Northern Africa. The
coloring property referred to as lawsone
comes from the center vein of the leaves,
and has a content of 1 percent to 5 percent
of red-orange molecules.

The leaves, which contain the highest concentration of color molecules, are crushed, finely powdered and sifted ... this becomes the product applied on the skin (body art) and hair.

The henna powder is combined with an acidic product such as lemon juice, orange juice or grapefruit juice to create a paste – thorough mixing is important for the proper development of color.

Henna, also know as **vegetable dye,** is not always encouraged to be used in a salon due to the length of development time and the possibility of interfering with other chemical services.

"For more information about henna and how to use it, visit www.Mehandi.com."

Non-Professional Haircoloring

Metallic (me-tal-lic) or Progressive (pro-gres-sive) Dye products **contain metals that produce various colors.** This type of color **creates a slow progression of color** that occurs by a series of repeated color applications. The hair will gradually get darker, dull-looking and the color will appear unnatural. The type of metallic salts in the color formula determines the end color result on the hair. Some of the metal material used is copper, lead acetate, silver nitrate, iron salts or nickel.

These types of metallic color ingredients are typically found in store-bought haircolor products due to manufacturing and marketing of a less expensive color product.

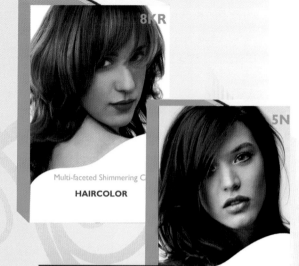

Multi-faceted Shimmering C
HAIRCOLOR

Multi-faceted Shimmering Color
HAIRCOLOR

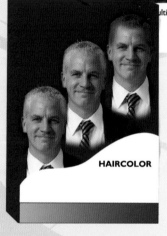

HAIRCOLOR

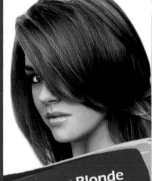

Copper Blonde

7K

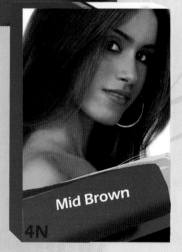

Mid Brown

4N

Compound (com-pound) Dyes are colors that **combine both metallic salts and henna to create the color formula.** Some manufacturers will even **add other chemical ingredients** such as paraphenylenediamine (para-phe-na-lyn-di-a-mine) to create a wider selection of colors. Compound dyes are very misleading to the consumer – not all the ingredients are listed depending on where the product was manufactured. When a commercial haircolor product advertises henna in various colors such as black or blonde, it is referred to as compound henna. **Compound hennas** consist of a **low-grade henna, metal salts and other chemical ingredients.**

NOTE: Any client/guest suspected of using a store-bought product must have a strand test to determine if metallic or compound dyes are on the hair.

Online Resources ...

Search the web for all kinds of beauty industry information, news, products, shows or even just to chat with your fellow artists.

Americas Beauty Show (ABS)
www.americasbeautyshow.com

Color Express® Inc.
www.colorexpress.org

Cosmoprof International
www.cosmoprof.com

Farouk Systems
www.farouk.com

Goldwell
www.goldwell-northamerica.com/site/products

International Beauty Show (IBS), New York
www.ibsnewyork.com

National Cosmetology Association (NCA)
www.salonprofessionals.org

Redken – Haircolor
www.redken.com/salon-services/haircolor

Renbow International – Haircolor Experts
www.renbow.co.uk

The Henna Page™
www.hennapage.com

Professional Beauty Association (PBA)
www.probeauty.org

Wella Professionals
www.wellausa.com

www.hair
search

"Hey, try to search your way to these haircoloring sites — most major haircolor manufacturers provide helpful information."

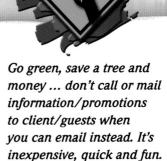

Go green, save a tree and money ... don't call or mail information/promotions to client/guests when you can email instead. It's inexpensive, quick and fun.

Haircoloring Tools ...

COLOR BRUSH AND BOWL

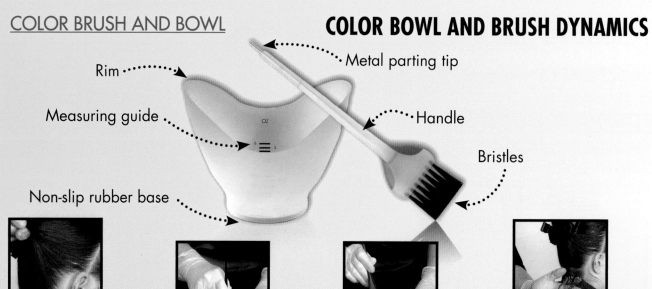

Rim

Metal parting tip

Measuring guide

Handle

Bristles

Non-slip rubber base

COLOR BOWL AND BRUSH DYNAMICS

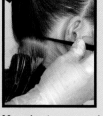

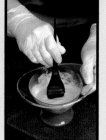

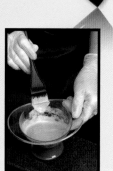

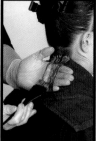

Use plastic or metal tip of brush handle to part a ¼ inch (0.6 cm) subsection of hair.

Place bristles of brush into color mixture.

Swipe opposite side of brush on edge of bowl to remove excess color mixture from bristles.

Hold subsection of hair with opposite hand and place bristles onto subsection of hair. Cover subsection of hair according to color procedure being performed.

APPLICATOR BOTTLE

Nozzle tip

Bottle

Nozzle tip

APPLICATOR BOTTLE DYNAMICS

Measuring guide

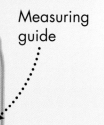

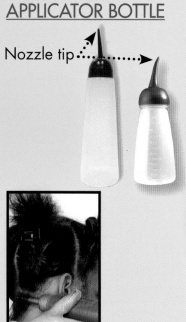

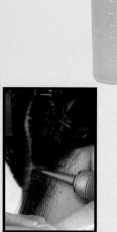

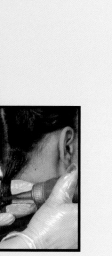

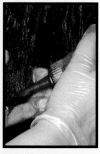

Use nozzle tip to part a ¼ inch (0.6 cm) subsection of hair.

Place nozzle tip at scalp along parting. Squeeze out the amount of color needed for accurate coverage.

Use nozzle tip to spread color along subsection of hair. Continue to place color onto subsection of hair.

Cover entire subsection to the hair ends.

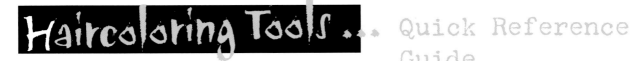

Haircoloring Tools ... Quick Reference Guide

HAIRCOLOR CAP AND HOOK

HAIRCOLOR CAP AND HOOK DYNAMICS

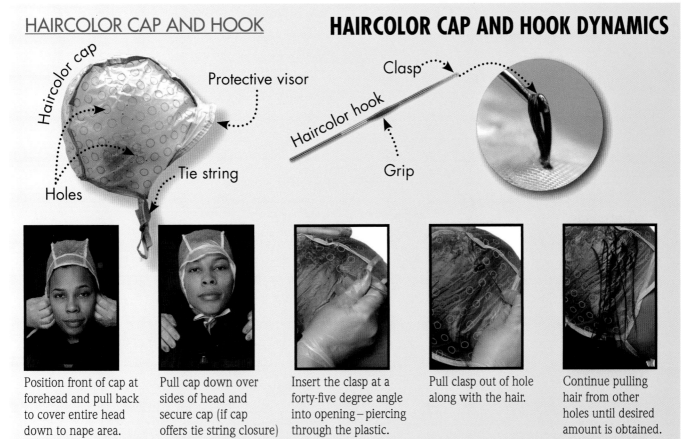

Haircolor cap

Protective visor

Clasp

Haircolor hook

Grip

Tie string

Holes

Position front of cap at forehead and pull back to cover entire head down to nape area.

Pull cap down over sides of head and secure cap (if cap offers tie string closure) to create a snug fit.

Insert the clasp at a forty-five degree angle into opening – piercing through the plastic.

Pull clasp out of hole along with the hair.

Continue pulling hair from other holes until desired amount is obtained.

HAIRCOLORING FOIL

HAIRCOLORING FOIL DYNAMICS

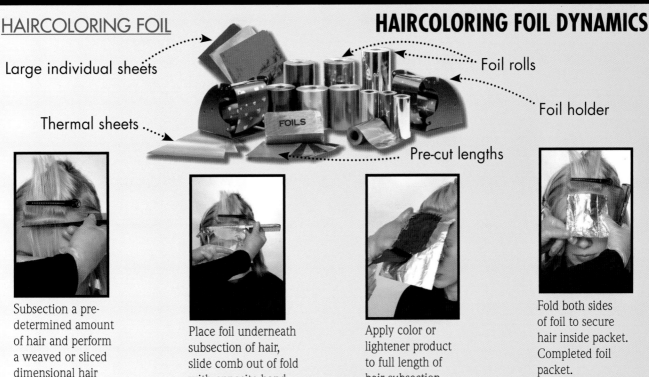

Large individual sheets

Foil rolls

Foil holder

Thermal sheets

FOILS

Pre-cut lengths

Subsection a pre-determined amount of hair and perform a weaved or sliced dimensional hair technique.

Place foil underneath subsection of hair, slide comb out of fold with opposite hand holding hair and foil in place.

Apply color or lightener product to full length of hair subsection – fold foil in half.

Fold both sides of foil to secure hair inside packet. Completed foil packet.

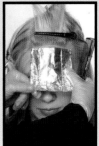

Chapter 2 • HAIRCOLORING TOOLS

59

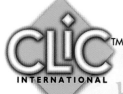
Haircoloring Tools **REVIEW QUESTIONS**

FILL-IN-THE-BLANKS

A.	**Air Purification System**
B.	**Applicator Bottle**
C.	**Chemical Aprons**
D.	**Coloring Combs**
E.	**Color Key**
F.	**Compound**
G.	**Developer**
H.	**Filler**
I.	**Haircolor Brushes**
J.	**Haircolor Cap**
K.	**Haircoloring Foil**
L.	**Henna**
M.	**Hydrometer**
N.	**Liquid Hydrogen Peroxide**
O.	**Mascara**
P.	**Permanent Haircolor**
Q.	**Protective Cream**
R.	**Robes**
S.	**Semi-Permanent Haircolor**
T.	**Toner**

1. _____ dyes combine both metallic salts and low-grade henna.

2. _____ is inserted at end of the color tube to remove color.

3. _____ are worn by the customer/guest during the haircolor service to eliminate clothing damage.

4. _____ isolates sections of hair being colored from the remaining hair that is not receiving color.

5. _____ is a deposit-only color and penetrates into the cuticle layer of the hair.

6. _____ contains holes in which a pre-determined amount of hair is pulled to be colored of lightened.

7. _____ are worn by the professional to protect clothing from chemical damage and stains during all hair services.

8. _____ perform a neat and accurate application of color or lightener on the hair.

9. _____ are used to create the weaving and slicing techniques with foil placement.

10. _____ is an instrument that measures the strength (volumes) of hydrogen peroxide.

11. _____ is considered a form of temporary color.

12. _____ is a pastel or light level of haircolor placed on pre-lightened hair.

13. _____ is another name for hydrogen peroxide, which is mixed with haircolor and lightener.

14. _____ holds low viscosity types of color or lightener.

15. _____ is available to clean the air within the salon.

16. _____ is applied along client/guest's hairline prior to haircolor application.

17. _____ is a pure, natural form of red-orange color.

18. _____ is the form of H_2O_2 used to test its strength in a hydrometer.

19. _____ penetrates into cuticle and cortex layers and lasts until new hair growth appears.

20. _____ is used to equalize the porosity in the cuticle layer of the hair shaft.

STUDENT'S NAME   DATE   GRADE

color
elements
intensity
molecules
pH
primary
vivid

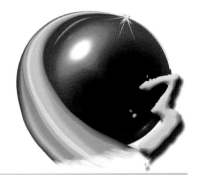

Science
of Haircoloring

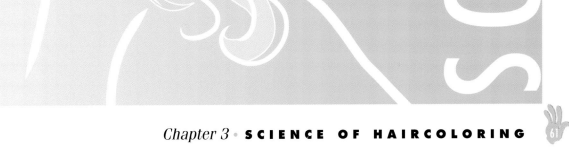

SCIENCE

Origin of Light ...

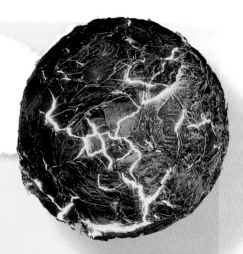

According to scientific research, it all started more than 13 billion years ago, with "The Big Bang Theory."

Radiation whirled into an expanding sphere called the **"Primordial Fireball."** After thousands of years, the fireball cooled, and left behind a giant heap of matter. That matter gradually broke apart to form the galaxies, stars and planets within our solar system.

Then, approximately 5 billion years ago, light was born!

A cloud of hydrogen and helium mixed with dust began to contract under the forces of its own gravity. This contraction generated so much heat that nuclear reactions began converting all of the hydrogen to helium. That **cloud became known as our sun**, and it has been shining steadily ever since, illuminating and enriching our earth with beautiful and vibrant colors!

"Wow! If we didn't have the sun, we wouldn't have light and if we didn't have light, there would not be any color ... truly amazing!"

Origin of Light ..

You are about to embark on the journey of lifelong learning with regard to haircolor. We are fortunate to have a legacy of information and knowledge from the brilliant scientists and researchers who came before us.

In 420 BCE when scientific inquiry and investigation was in its early stages, the **Greek philosopher Democritus** (De-moc-ri-tus) declared, "The only existing things are atoms and empty space – all else is mere opinion."

2,100 years later, **Sir Isaac Newton** made a very important contribution to science with his discovery of the color spectrum, yet he still did not know the true nature of light. For the next 250 years, scientists and philosophers continued their quest to unravel the many mysteries of energy, light and matter. It was **Albert Einstein who pulled everything together into one extraordinary discovery – relativity.** Through his Theory of Relativity, Einstein left us with the puzzling revelation that light, energy and matter are all one and the same!

Democritus

Can you imagine the implications of that discovery, and what an awesome universe we live in? There are many, many galaxies, trillions of stars and a vast expanse of space filled with electromagnetic waves. These waves, like parcels of energy, originate from the stars and the sun.

Albert Einstein

Origin of Light ...

What is Light?

Light is a form of energy that travels in invisible waves, much like radio waves, x-rays and microwaves. Light rays carry photons (fo-ton), which are little packets of energy that stimulate light-sensitive cells in our eyes so that we can see. Light waves travel very rapidly – at a rate of more than 186,000 miles per second – making them the fastest traveling waves in the universe.

In 1676, Sir Isaac Newton discovered the connection between light and color during his famous prism experiment. He found that when **light is projected through a prism, it splits into The Visible Spectrum of Light:** red, orange, yellow, green, blue, indigo **and** violet, also known as chromatic colors. He also found that if those color beams are redirected through another prism, they will reunite back to their original form of white light.

This phenomenon can be viewed in nature by the breathtaking beauty of a rainbow. The rainbow is created by exactly the same splitting of light that Newton discovered. Billions of miniature prisms are created by water droplets in the air. When sunlight is filtered through those water droplets, The Visible Spectrum of Light appears in the form of a rainbow. Our old friend **Mr. Roy G. Biv** can help you remember all the colors of the spectrum of light by using the letters in his name ...

Red
Orange
Yellow
Green
Blue
Indigo
Violet

Sir Isaac Newton

"A physics professor, Alan Kostelecky of Indiana University, describes light as 'a shimmering of ever-present vectors in empty space' and compares it to waves across a field of grain!"

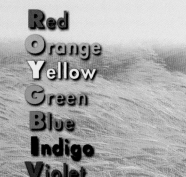

Theory of Color ...

Haircoloring is the science and art of changing the color of the hair by placing artificial color or lightener on the hair. When applying color on the hair, a **professional must have knowledge of the color wheel and the law of color** in order to produce the best complementary color results.

Color brightens our world and captivates our eyes. It is a physical phenomenon of light or visual perception associated with the various wavelengths seen by the eye. Color has meaning; reaction to color is either logical or emotional, varying from one individual to another.

All color is derived from the primary colors and the tool that best describes this is the color wheel. The color wheel is used as a support for the law of color to visually prove how all colors are created.

For the cosmetologist, the law of color provides a unique understanding of color formulation, which artists have tested and proven many times over. All color begins with the three basic primary colors!

RED

YELLOW

BLUE

"Light is color when projected through a prism ... proven by Sir Isaac Newton!"

Principles of Color ...

The Three Main Principles of Color

Primary colors are the **basic colors** from which all other colors are produced. These colors are also considered the **purest** colors. They are red, yellow and blue.

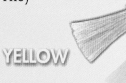

Secondary colors are formed when **combining two primary colors in equal proportions.** The combinations of the following primary colors will give you the secondary colors: Red + Yellow = Orange, Yellow + Blue = Green, Red + Blue = Violet

Tertiary colors are created by **mixing a primary color with the neighboring secondary color.** They are red-orange, red-violet, yellow-orange, yellow-green, blue-green and blue-violet. Tertiary colors always state the primary color first.

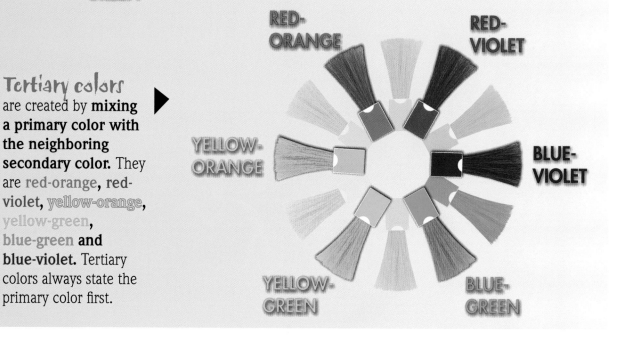

Principles of Color ...

Complementary colors are used to remove undesirable colors or undertones in the hair. They are derived from mixing a primary and a secondary color that are situated opposite each other on the color wheel.

Example: **Blue and Orange (Y & R), Red and Green (Y & B), Yellow and Violet (R & B).**

These colors when mixed together will **cancel out the undesirable color.** For example, if you want to neutralize a green cast or undertone, add **red**, which is found opposite the green on the color wheel. Red is the missing primary color needed that will **neutralize** or counteract the green. Other color combinations that neutralize each other are: **blue** and **orange, yellow and violet.** When combining complementary colors, each color must be of equal strength and value in order to achieve the desired result.

RED

ORANGE

VIOLET

YELLOW

BLUE

GREEN

NOTE: When adding any secondary color to its primary, the result is a combination of all three primary colors.

Neutral colors are not located within the visible light spectrum and contain minimal to no pigment or color. These colors are white, black and gray and exist through either the reflection or absorption of light.

- **White** occurs when **all colors are reflected** at an equal distance.

- **Black** appears when **all the colors are absorbed** equally, reflecting no color.

- **Gray** is a result of **partial color reflection.** The lightness to darkness of gray is determined by the amount of light reflection. When a greater amount of light is reflected, the result is light gray; a small amount of gray reflected results in dark gray.

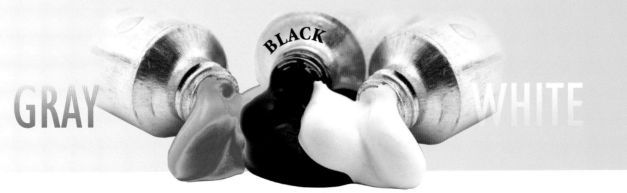

GRAY   BLACK   WHITE

The Law of Color ...

The Law of Color provides an understanding of the relationships of color that have been tested and proven. The Law of Color begins with the basics, which are the purest colors of blue, red and yellow.

◀ Blue

Blue is a **cool color.** When adding blue to a haircolor mixture, you are adding **darkness, cool tones and depth.** In the cortex layer of the hair, blue pigments are located **closest to the surface and leave the hair first** during permanent haircolor development.

Red ▶

Red is a **warm color.** When adding red to a haircolor mixture, you are adding **warmth and richness.** Red pigments are located **deep within the cortex layer of the hair and are difficult to remove** during permanent haircolor development.

◁ Yellow

Yellow is also a **warm color.** When adding yellow to a haircolor mixture, you are adding **light and brightness.** Yellow pigments are found **deepest within the hair shaft** and are the **most difficult to remove** during permanent haircolor development without significant damage to the hair.

The Law of Color ..

WHITE

BLACK

BROWN

Mixing the pigments of the three primary colors in equal proportions will result in the color black. White is the absence of pigments. Brown is a combination of all three primaries, but in unequal proportions – three yellow, two red and one blue.

"Remember, practice makes perfect. Your client/guest's natural hair pigments will always combine with the haircoloring products used to affect the end color result. Through practice and experimentation, you will learn this balance."

Temperature of Color ...

COLOR HAS A TEMPERATURE

Color is classified into two temperatures or undertones: **Warm and Cool**

Undertone is the underlying or base color seen within the predominant color. It can be a result of the natural inborn pigments, or artificially created to produce a two-level effect.

Warm is associated with fire or the sun. Colors that include red, yellow or orange **are classified as being warm.**

Cool is associated with the sky or water. Colors ranging from green, **blue** and **violet** **are considered cool.**

Pure colors can usually be classified under the seasons of the year when related to their temperature of warm or cool. **Clear/cool** palettes are especially found in the **winter** and clear/warm palettes are generally found in the **spring.** You will find that most **summer colors are mute/cool** and **autumn colors are mute/warm** creating a soft or dusty feeling. To obtain cool colors, gray is added and to achieve warm colors, brown is added.

HAIRCOLORING

Elements of Color...

To recognize the art behind coloring hair, the cosmetologist will need to understand the elements of color. The artist will depend upon these elements to apply color basics, or to bring harmony to unbalanced face proportions. The elements of color are also necessary as the artist expands upon his or her creativity to create special effect hairdesigns, and to set the stage for the future haircolor trends.

Elements of Color are:
- Pigment
- Three Dimensions of a Color
- Color Harmonies

Disclaimer: *As you read the following information, keep in mind, it is to review the elements of color – not to be confused with haircolor formulating (that is discussed in Chapter 5).*

Pigment is what gives color its color. No matter what the pigment's source, whether natural, chemical or mineral, the same color theory holds true. All forms of haircolor contain pigments whether it is the color directly out of the bottle or color that requires oxidation to create the color result.

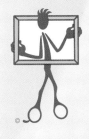

"Study the masters of art for inspiration. Visit your local museum!"

Three dimensions of a color, which help to accurately describe color are

1. Hue
2. Value
3. Intensity

1. Hue is a **general name for color.** It is determined by the wavelength's range within the light spectrum or **its position on the color wheel.** Each color has subtle variations; when viewing a color, the individual will decide the color name. Primary colors are the basis by which all other colors are established.

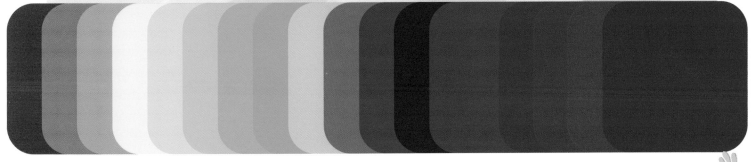

Elements of Color ...

2. Value is **evaluating the hue of a color** and determining whether it is **light or dark** due to the quantity of light reflected or absorbed. When a **hue reflects varying amounts of light, the wavelength is changed therefore the color is changed.** If the amount of light reflected is high resulting in less absorption, or if **white is mixed with the hue, the color will appear light** (for example: yellow). If a **minimal amount of light is reflected** as a result of more absorption, or if **black is mixed with the hue, the color will appear darker** (for example: blue). In the manufacturing of haircolor, value is usually referred to as level, which distinguishes between light, medium and dark colors.

Strawberry blonde

Red-orange

White

Auburn

Red-orange

Black

3. Intensity is the **strength of the color's appearance,** which is determined by the **hue's degree of saturation and purity of light reflection.** If there is **high clarity** in the reflection of light, **a bright, vivid color will result.** If there is **low clarity in light reflection, a dull, drab color** will appear. Mixing more then one color is another approach to altering intensity. By adding black or white to a color, it will become either darker or lighter therefore increasing or decreasing the intensity.
Example:
red-orange + white = strawberry blonde and red-orange + black = **auburn.**

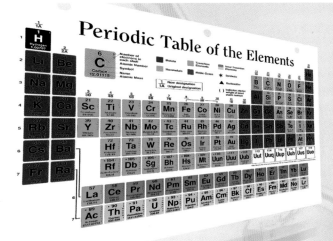

Periodic Table of the Elements

2. Element is any substance made of one type of atom and **cannot be broken down** into a simpler one chemically; it is a **basic unit of matter.** An element chart is used to identify each element with its symbol.

3. Molecule (mol-e-cule) is created when **one or more atoms combine** and retain their chemical and physical properties **to form matter.** Example: a molecule of water consists of two hydrogen atoms and one oxygen atom or an oxygen molecule consists of two oxygen atoms.

4. Compound, also known as **chemical compound,** is a chemical substance consisting of atoms or ions of two or more elements in definite proportions that **cannot be separated by physical means. Example:** molecules of water are considered chemical compounds because they consist of two different atoms, hydrogen and oxygen.

Chemical bonding occurs with the connection or linking of amino acids. Amino acids are chemical compounds that are made up of **hydrogen, oxygen, nitrogen, carbon and sulfur elements.** Amino acids need to come together to form the structure of hair (cortical layer).

Haircolor Chemistry ...

As haircolorists, we need to **understand what is in the bottle or tube of haircolor** *that is able to change the color of our hair. There are many ways we can alter our haircolor depending on the desired end result.* **Haircolor falls under four main categories: temporary, semi-permanent, demi-permanent and permanent.** *If needing a quick fix for a special occasion, a temporary color can be applied and then washed out within a couple of hours or even the next day –* **OR** *if the client/guest desires something more long-term, he or she can get a permanent color that would possibly last four to six weeks, until regrowth. The chemical composition for each category of color will be different so as to create varying types of color strengths as well as a multitude of shades/colors.*

NON-OXIDATIVE HAIRCOLORS:

Temporary color is made up of **large**, **direct dye (pre-colored) molecules** that are **unable to penetrate the hair** and therefore create only a physical change to the hair. These dye molecules are considered **certified and approved by the Food and Drug Administration (FDA).** When the hair is cleansed, the dye molecules are washed away along with the physical color change on the hair ... no chemical reaction occurs with temporary color.

1

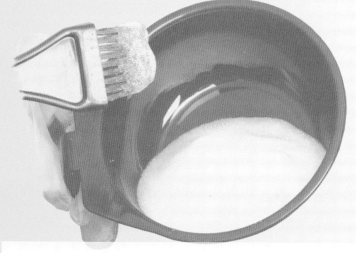

Temporary colors come in multiple forms such as liquid rinses, shampoos/conditioners, foams, sprays or styling lotions/gels ... even mascara and eyebrow pencils are considered temporary colors.

Disclaimer: *The information provided on these pages is a general overview of product. We highly recommend that you always read the manufacturer's instructions before handling any haircolor or hair lightener product.*

Haircolor Chemistry ...

Semi-Permanent color consists of both **large and small** direct dye molecules in which the small molecules will penetrate the cuticle and the large molecules will coat the hair surface.

Some manufacturers will add alkaline agents, solvents and/or surfactants along with the large and small dye molecules to **enhance the color longevity** on the hair. **No chemical reaction occurs** with semi-permanent color – the color in the bottle is the color that goes on the hair. This type of color **gradually fades** – resulting in **NO "line of demarcation"** and color lasts beyond the client/guest's daily hair cleansing.

Semi-permanent color is also an excellent choice if a client/guest's existing natural or artificial haircolor needs to be **enriched or refreshed,** or even if he or she wants to **add a gloss or shine** to the hair.

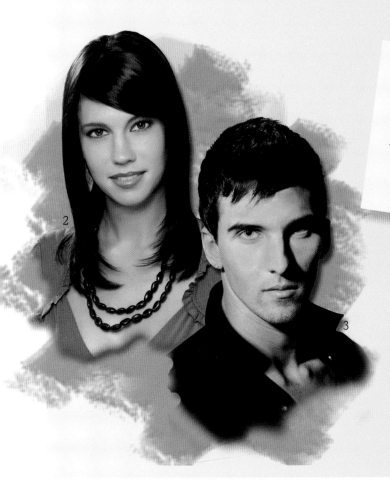

SEMI-PERMANENT

1

NOTE: How each of these colors affect the hair will be discussed in the Biological Powers chapter.

2

3

"Temporary and semi-permanent colors are considered non-oxidative because no chemical mixing or reaction takes place to produce these colors on the hair. The color in the bottle is what you will see on the hair."

The next two categories of haircolor involve the chemical process called **OXIDATION.**

Oxidation (ox-i-da-tion) is the **chemical reaction** that occurs when oxygen is released from a substance. This reaction assists in the **development of color** on the hair. The **oxidizing agent, hydrogen peroxide,** is mixed with the haircolor (cream, gel, liquid, etc.), which produces the oxidation, creating the new end color result. Oxidation is **increased when using a high (30) volume or percentage of hydrogen peroxide** and the opposite will occur when the color formulation contains a **low (10) volume or percentage of hydrogen peroxide**, resulting in a **decrease in oxidation.** To obtain an equal balance of oxidation, use 20 volume or percentage H_2O_2, which is the most commonly used volume by cosmetologists.

OXIDATIVE HAIRCOLORS:

Demi-Permanent color, sometimes referred to as **long-lasting semi-permanent color,** contains **small indirect or combination of direct and indirect dye molecules,** which are mixed with a **low volume (4 to 7) or percentage of hydrogen peroxide.** This formula creates a slow oxidation, which enables further penetration of the color molecules into the cuticle and partially the cortex of the hair, creating a long-lasting color.

1

DEMI-PERMANENT

Permanent color, commonly known as **aniline derivative** (an-i-line de-riv-a-tive) **tint**, is made up of small colorless molecules that have varying grades or amounts of ammonia. The colorless molecules, also known as **paraphenylenediamine** (para-phen-nil-ene-di-a-mine) or **para dyes**, turn color once the oxidation process takes place. The colorless molecules must be **mixed with hydrogen peroxide** in order to efficiently produce the colored molecules needed to give hair its artificial color. This is the strongest category of haircolor due to its ability to penetrate into the cortex of the hair, creating longevity of color.

PERMANENT

1

2

NOTE: The term **"tint"** is sometimes used to describe permanent color. **Tint** is defined as a color shade or hair dye that provides color.

Chemistry of Haircolor Ingredients ...

Permanent haircolor can produce a **wide range of colors as well as last longer** than any other category of haircolor. Responsible for the strength of this color is the addition of other chemical ingredients that assist in the color's penetration of the cuticle and cortex of the hair. Hair lighteners also may contain this common ingredient.

Ammonia

Ammonia (am-mo-nia) is a compound made up of **one nitrogen atom and three hydrogen atoms (NH_3)** that quickly evaporate. It is an alkaline substance that **emits a gaseous odor** (strong and unpleasant) and is used in the manufacturing of haircolor and hair lightening. The amount of ammonia in a bottle (or tube) of color is gradually decreased or increased in strength to **produce various levels of haircolor.** The ammonia's high pH level assists with the color's chemical process to raise the cuticle scales, which will then help the color or lightener to penetrate the hair.

Alkanolamines (al-kan-ol-am-eenz) are other types of **alkalizing agents** used in the manufacturing of haircolors or lighteners. They are large, organic molecules that are soluble in water, and have **little to no odor,** and therefore are beneficial when used to **replace the ammonia in some haircolors or lighteners.**

Some examples of alkanolamines are **aminomethyl propanol or AMP** (a-mee-no-meth-yl pro-pan-ol) and **monoethanolamine or MEA** (ma-no-eth-an-ol-am-een), which are formed from the chemical reaction of ammonia and ethylene oxide. Keep in mind that alkanolamines might not have the same processing results as ammonia due to a different chemical breakdown.

Activator is a powder or crystal form of an **oxidizing agent and/or persulfates** (per-sul-fates), which are salts taken from persulfuric acid. Activators are packaged in small quantities to be mixed with the existing lightener or color formulation to **increase the strength of the oxidation process.** Some other commonly used names for activator are accelerator, booster, intensifier or protinator.

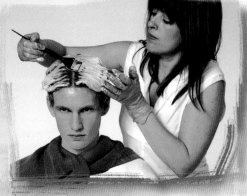

Hair Lightener Chemistry...

Hair Lightener, sometimes referred to as **bleach or decolorizer,** is a **combination of hydrogen peroxide with an ammonia agent** or other type of alkalizing agents. The objective of the lightener is to **diffuse the natural melanin or artificial pigments** in the hair to lighten the existing melanin and create a light haircolor (blonde).

Diffuse is defined as – **to spread apart or scatter** over a certain area, allowing **light to reflect through.** The scattering of melanin or pigment in the hair allows light reflection instead of absorption, which will produce lighter haircolors.

If the desired level of color is unable to be reached with permanent haircolor, then a hair lightener is used. The strong alkaline nature of the **ammonia or alkanolamines activates the hydrogen peroxide** creating the oxidation process and therefore speeding up the decolorization of the melanin or pigment in the hair.

Lightener is available in three forms: oil, cream and powder.

- **Oil and cream lighteners** are both safe and effective for any **on-the-scalp hair services.** They both **must be mixed with hydrogen peroxide; however,** the cream lightener consists of conditioning or thickening agents that add **viscosity** as opposed to the oil lightener, which is more liquid. Cream lighteners may require the addition of an activator to increase its oxidizing strength.

- **Powder lighteners** contain persulfate salts (same as in the activators) and **must be mixed with hydrogen peroxide** to activate the oxidation process and/or decolorization. A powder lightener is generally considered stronger and fast-acting and is meant for only **off-the-scalp hair services** such as highlighting. Some powder lighteners contain pigments to assist in neutralizing unwanted color tones that may appear during the decolorization process.

LIGHTENERS

Hydrogen Peroxide Chemistry...

Hydrogen Peroxide contains molecules consisting of **two hydrogen atoms and two oxygen atoms (H_2O_2).** Substitute names for H_2O_2 are **developer, catalyst or oxidizing agent.** Hydrogen peroxide has an acidic solution with a pH ranging from 2.5 to 4 that is produced in volumes or percentages, which are distinguished by a number such as **10, 20, 30 or 40. Volume** means **percentage of oxygen gas released** from the hydrogen peroxide. The 10, 20, 30 and 40 volumes are used for permanent color development, with 30 and 40 volumes typically used for high-lift haircoloring. **Forty volume H_2O_2 is not recommended for lightener application unless it is an off-the-scalp service.** Follow manufacturer's directions before mixing any haircolor or lightener products. Refer to chart for the hydrogen peroxide volume with its percentage of oxygen gas to water.

Hydrogen Peroxide Volume	Percentage of Oxygen Gas	Percentage of water
10 Volume	3%	97%
20 Volume	6%	94%
30 Volume	9%	91%
40 Volume	12%	88%

NOTE: Think of hydrogen peroxide being much like water (H_2O), but containing one extra oxygen atom. That one extra atom assists in the oxidation and decolorizing of melanin in haircoloring and lightening services.

Hydrogen Peroxide Chemistry ...

Hydrogen peroxide is manufactured in a **cream form** that creates a thick viscosity when mixing the color formulation. This cream developer is made up of creaming agents such as alkanolamines (al·kan·all·am·eenz) and fatty alcohols. This form of hydrogen peroxide no longer appears clear, like water, but has an **opaque appearance.**

Hydrogen peroxide is an unstable chemical, which means it can **deteriorate quickly if in contact with heat, dirt, light, metal** or any other contaminates. The **proper storage of H$_2$O$_2$** is to keep it in its original container and place in a cool, dry and dark area. **DO NOT place any unused peroxide** back into the original container in order to prevent contamination.

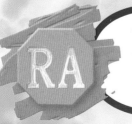

"Refer to chapter 5 for reducing (diluting) the strength of hydrogen peroxide."

CAUTION: Any oxidizing agent is considered potentially hazardous to the skin, lungs and eyes; possibly causing skin burning and damage. Be sure to wear gloves, safety glasses and dust mask when working around an oxidizing agent ... refer to the MSDS and manufacturer's instructions for safety and handling of any product.

pH

*A*wareness *of pH will further your knowledge on the strength of haircolor and hair lightener and its effects on the hair and skin. This will increase the professional's awareness in using safe reliable products, which will pose no risk to your client/guest's health and well-being.*

Potential Hydrogen (pH) is the concentrated potential amount of hydrogen ions in a solution containing water. The term pH is derived from the **Danish word "potenz" hydrogen or "hydrogen strength."**

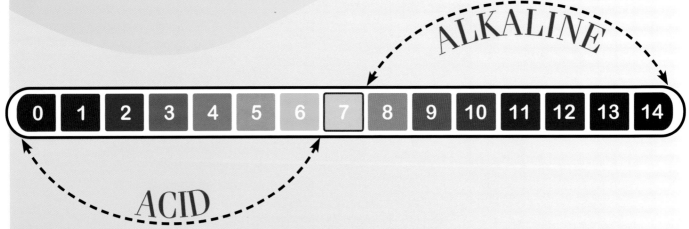

ALKALINE

0 1 2 3 4 5 6 7 8 9 10 11 12 13 14

ACID

Acidic solutions contain more hydrogen ions and **alkaline** (also known as **base**) solutions contain a smaller amount of hydrogen ions. **Acidic products contract and harden hair, and have a sour taste. Alkaline products soften and swell hair, and have a bitter taste.** A solution tested using the **pH scale** will show a range from **0 to 14.** This scale shows the dramatic increase in acidity or alkalinity when moving from one end of the pH scale to the other.

ACID	NEUTRAL	ALKALINE
pH ranges from 0 to 6.9	pH is 7	pH ranges from 7.1 to 14

0   1   2   3   4   5   6   7   8   9   10   11   12   13   14

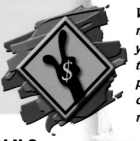

When you understand how to maintain proper hair pH levels, you will be able to market the most suitable and safe professional products to the customer/guest for use as home maintenance treatments.

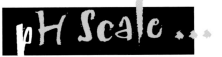

pH Scale ...

The pH scale was conceived in 1909 by the **Danish biochemist Soren Peter Lauritz Sorenson.** He realized that water was balanced with an equal amount of positive hydrogen ions (H+) and negative hydroxide ions (OH). **The amount of hydrogen ion concentrations are measured** to determine if a solution is acid, neutral or alkaline.

The pH scale is designed logarithmically, meaning each number on the pH scale represents an **increase in multiples of 10**. Therefore, each number on the scale is 10 times more alkaline or acidic than the next number in the sequence ... from **neutral 7 up for alkalinity** and from **neutral 7 down for acidity.**

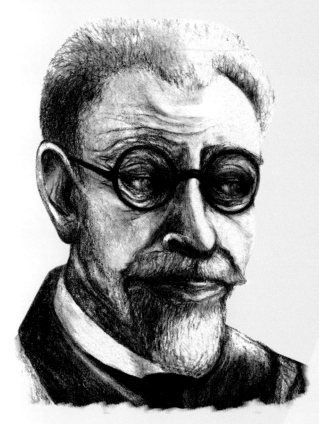

Soren Peter Lauritz Sorenson

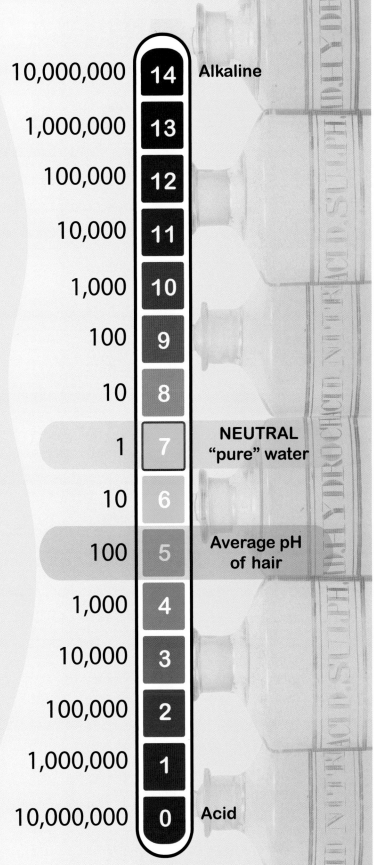

10,000,000	14	Alkaline
1,000,000	13	
100,000	12	
10,000	11	
1,000	10	
100	9	
10	8	
1	7	NEUTRAL "pure" water
10	6	
100	5	Average pH of hair
1,000	4	
10,000	3	
100,000	2	
1,000,000	1	
10,000,000	0	Acid

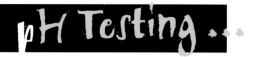

The **natural pH level of hair** ranges from **pH 4.5 to 5.5;** therefore, any hair products a professional uses should be **designed within the same pH range** for client/guest safety, comfort and reliability. Keep in mind, in order to achieve permanent hair textures and haircolors, chemicals are required to obtain the desired appearance. It is the finishing liquid tools such as shampoo, conditioner and styling aids that should be chosen for compatibility and restoring the hair back to its natural pH level.

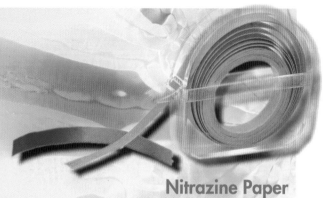

Nitrazine Paper

To determine if a product is within the natural hair pH range (4.5 to 5.5), or if it is low in acidity/high in alkalinity, test with small strips of color-coded **litmus** or **nitrazine paper.** These papers are the most widely used pH testing tool within the cosmetology industry.

Product Testing using pH Papers:

NOTE: Always read manufacturer's instructions for the safety and handling of all pH testing tools.

Litmus Paper

Litmus pH paper – immerse paper into product. If paper turns **blue**, product is alkaline; if paper turns **red**, product is acid.

Nitrazine pH paper – immerse paper into product, wait 30 seconds. Color of paper can range from orange to **dark purple**. Use the color chart that is packaged with the nitrazine paper and compare the immersed paper against the charted color, which will decide the product's pH number.

Other pH testing methods are pH pencil and pH meter.

pH pencil

- The **pH pencil** is an alternative tool for testing all liquid products. When testing, moisten a small area on a clean surface(glass or porcelain) with the product. Use the **pH pencil to draw a line through the wet area** and wait about 15 seconds for color to appear. Use the accompanying color chart to determine the pH reading.

- The **pH meter unit** has an **electrode, which is submerged into an aqueous (water) solution,** which will display an accurate digital pH reading on the number scale located on the meter's unit.

pH meter

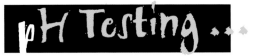

The following examples indicate the pH ranges of haircoloring products:

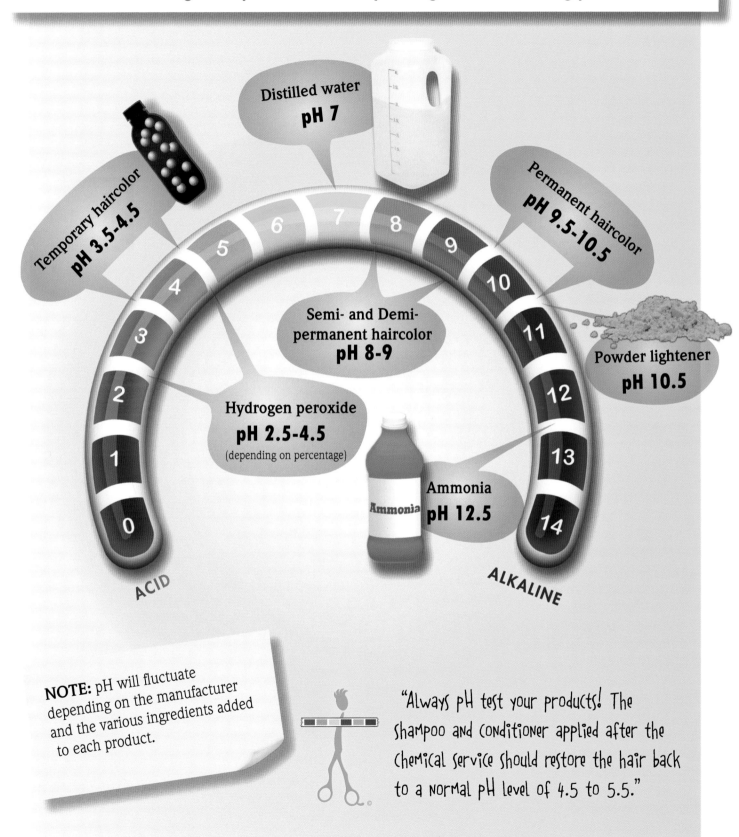

Distilled water
pH 7

Temporary haircolor
pH 3.5-4.5

Permanent haircolor
pH 9.5-10.5

Semi- and Demi-
permanent haircolor
pH 8-9

Powder lightener
pH 10.5

Hydrogen peroxide
pH 2.5-4.5
(depending on percentage)

Ammonia
pH 12.5

ACID

ALKALINE

NOTE: pH will fluctuate depending on the manufacturer and the various ingredients added to each product.

"Always pH test your products! The shampoo and conditioner applied after the chemical service should restore the hair back to a normal pH level of 4.5 to 5.5."

Chapter 3 • **SCIENCE OF HAIRCOLORING** 89

LAW OF COLOR

Primary colors

are the **basic colors** from which all other colors are produced. These colors are also considered the **purest** colors.

Secondary colors

are formed when **combining two primary colors** in equal proportions.

Tertiary colors

are created by **mixing a primary color with the neighboring secondary color.**

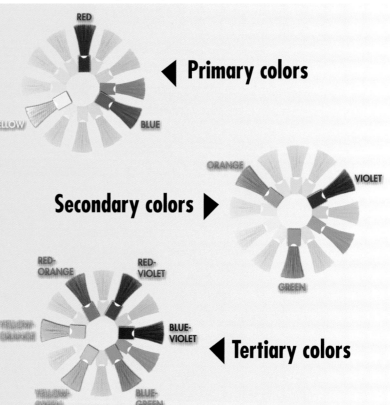

◀ **Primary colors**

Secondary colors ▶

◀ **Tertiary colors**

TEMPERATURE OF COLOR

Color is classified into two temperatures or undertones: **Warm and Cool**

Warm is associated with fire or the sun. Colors that include red, yellow and orange are classified as being warm.

Cool is associated with the sky or water. Colors ranging from green, blue and **violet** are considered cool.

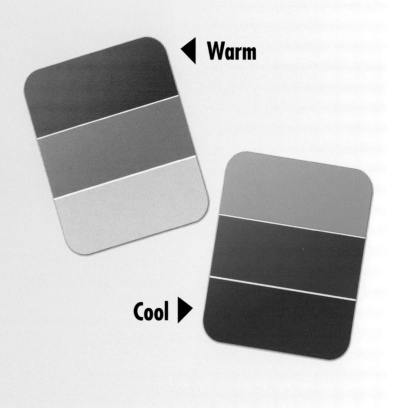

◀ **Warm**

Cool ▶

NON-OXIDATIVE HAIRCOLOR

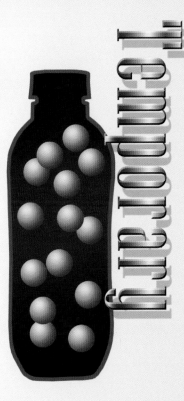

TEMPORARY COLOR

Temporary color is made up of large, **direct dye (pre-colored) molecules** that are unable to penetrate the hair and therefore create only a physical change to the hair. These dye molecules are considered **certified and approved by the Food and Drug Administration (FDA).** When the hair is cleansed, the dye molecules are washed away along with the physical color change on the hair ... no chemical reaction occurs with temporary color.

SEMI-PERMANENT COLOR

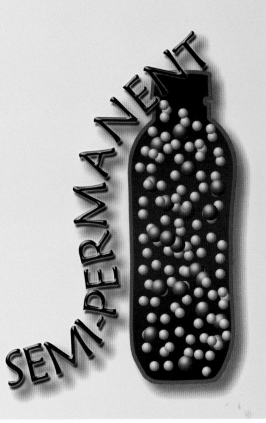

Semi-Permanent color consists of both large and **small direct dye molecules** in which the small molecules will penetrate the cuticle and the large molecules will coat the hair surface. No chemical reaction occurs with semi permanent color – the color in the bottle is the color that goes on the hair. This type of color gradually fades – resulting in NO "line of demarcation" and color lasts beyond the client/guest's daily hair cleansing.

OXIDATIVE HAIRCOLOR

DEMI-PERMANENT COLOR

Demi-Permanent color, sometimes referred to as **long-lasting semi-permanent color,** contains **small indirect or combination of direct and indirect dye molecules,** which are mixed with a **low volume (4 to 7) of hydrogen peroxide.** This formula creates a slow oxidation, which enables further penetration of the color molecules into the cuticle and partially the cortex of the hair, creating a long-lasting color.

PERMANENT COLOR

Permanent color, commonly known as **aniline derivative** (an-i-line de-riv-a-tive) **tint,** is made up of small colorless molecules that have varying grades or amounts of ammonia. The colorless molecules, also known as paraphenylenediamine (para-phen-nil-ene-di-a-mine) or para dyes, turn to a color once the oxidation process takes place.

The colorless molecules must be **mixed with hydrogen peroxide** in order to efficiently produce the colored molecules needed to give hair its artificial color. This is the strongest category of haircolor due to its ability to penetrate into the cortex of the hair, creating longevity of color.

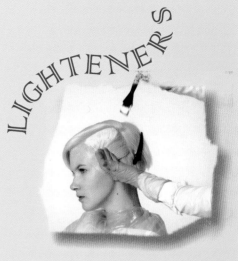

HAIR LIGHTENER

Hair Lightener, sometimes referred to as **bleach or decolorizer,** is a combination of hydrogen peroxide with an ammonia agent or other type of alkalizing agents. The objective of the lightener is to **diffuse the natural melanin or artificial pigments in the hair** to lighten the existing melanin and create a light haircolor (blonde). The strong alkaline nature of the ammonia or alkanolamines activates the hydrogen peroxide creating the oxidation process and therefore speeding up the decolorization of the melanin or pigment in the hair.

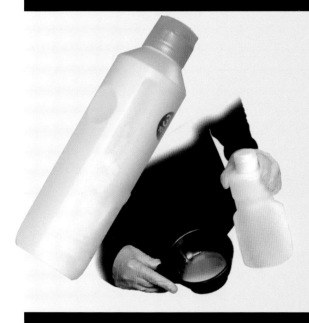

HYDROGEN PEROXIDE

Hydrogen Peroxide (hy-dro-gen per-ox-ide) contains molecules consisting of two hydrogen atoms and two oxygen atoms (H_2O_2). Substitute names for H_2O_2 are **developer, catalyst or oxidizing agent.** Hydrogen peroxide has an acidic solution with a pH ranging from 2.5 to 4 that is produced in volumes or percentages, which are distinguished by a number such as 10, 20, 30 or 40.

pH

Potential Hydrogen (pH) is the concentrated amount of hydrogen ions in a solution containing water. **Acidic solutions** contain more hydrogen ions and **alkaline solutions** contain a smaller amount of hydrogen ions. Acidic products **contract and harden hair,** and have a sour taste. Alkaline products **soften and swell hair,** and have a bitter taste. A solution tested using the **pH scale will show a range from 0 to 14.**

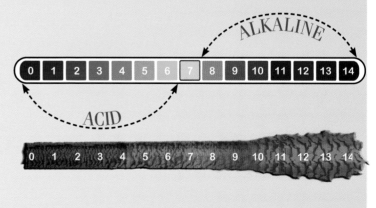

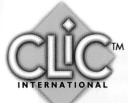

REVIEW QUESTIONS

MULTIPLE CHOICE

1. Who discovered the connection between light and color with his famous prism experiment?
   A. Albert Einstein
   B. Sir Isaac Newton
   C. Democritus

2. Which color is considered to have a warm temperature?
   A. orange
   B. blue
   C. red-violet

3. Which category of haircolor creates **ONLY** a physical change to the hair?
   A. temporary
   B. demi-permanent
   C. permanent

4. What is formed by combining one or more atoms?
   A. ion
   B. element
   C. molecule

5. What is the natural pH level of hair?
   A. 7
   B. 5.5 to 6
   C. 4.5 to 5.5

6. Blue-violet is considered which principle of color?
   A. primary
   B. secondary
   C. tertiary

7. What do alkaline products do to the hair?
   A. harden
   B. soften
   C. contract

8. The Visible Spectrum of Light consists of red, orange, yellow, green, blue, indigo and?
   A. pink
   B. violet
   C. gray

9. What color appears when all colors of the light spectrum are absorbed equally?
   A. black
   B. gray
   C. white

10. Which dimension of color determines the amount of light reflected or absorbed?
    A. hue
    B. value
    C. harmony

11. What is the chemical symbol for ammonia?
    A. H_2O_2
    B. H_2O
    C. NH_3

12. Which category of haircolor is mixed with hydrogen peroxide to assist in color development?
    A. temporary
    B. semi-permanent
    C. permanent

13. Which pH testing paper turns a range of colors, from orange to dark purple?
    A. nitrazine
    B. litmus
    C. sand

14. Which principle of color consists of the purest colors?
    A. primary
    B. secondary
    C. complementary

15. What is the general name for color?
    A. pigment
    B. hue
    C. light

16. What is the name of the positive charged particles found in the atom's nucleus?
    A. neutrons
    B. protons
    C. electrons

17. The category of haircolor that contains both large and small dye molecules is?
    A. demi-permanent
    B. semi-permanent
    C. temporary

18. What is the number range on the pH scale when a product tests acid?
    A. 7.1 to 14
    B. 7
    C. 0 to 6.9

19. What is another name for hydrogen peroxide?
    A. developer
    B. hue
    C. molecule

20. When pH tested, which product is considered high in alkalinity?
    A. ammonia
    B. hydrogen peroxide
    C. distilled water

STUDENT'S NAME   DATE   GRADE

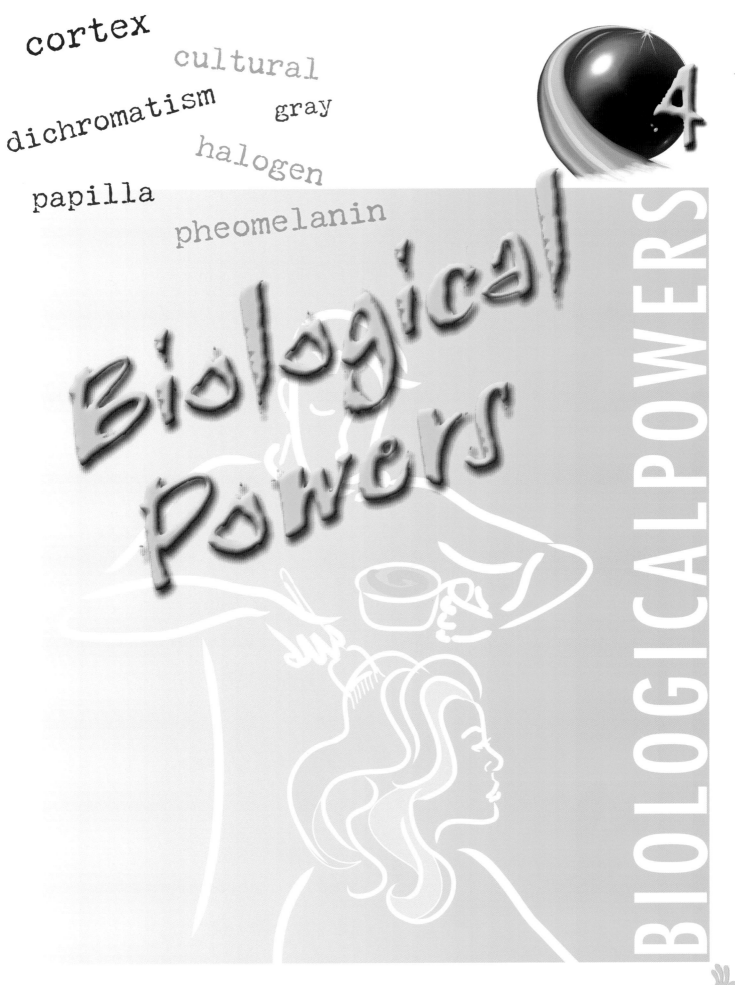

cortex

cultural

dichromatism   gray

halogen

papilla

pheomelanin

Biological Powers

BIOLOGICALPOWERS

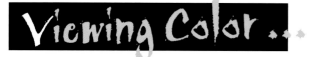

Light strikes an object and that object becomes

ILLUMINATED!

The **illuminated** object is captured by the human eye, processed and then transferred to our brains into a message.

This message is transformed, which allows us to experience the visual beauty of life that surrounds us every day!

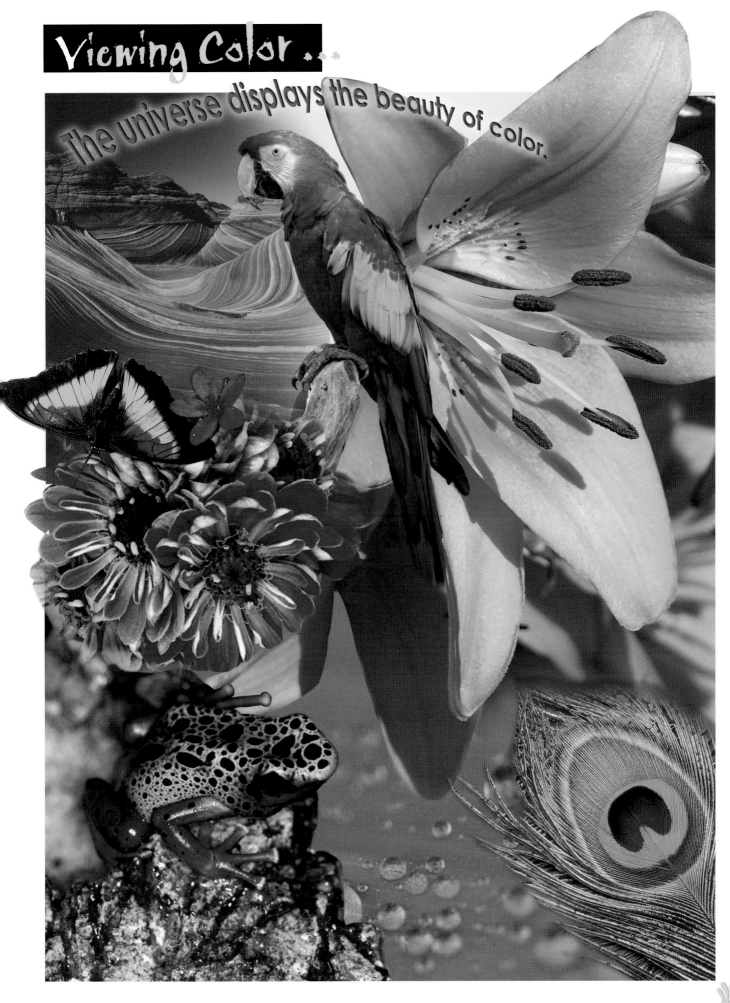

Viewing Color ...

The universe displays the beauty of color.

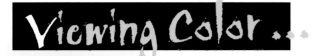

How do we see color?

It is well known that we **see with our eyes and think with our brains.** This seems so simple, but actually a complex process is involved when we look at objects. Within a fraction of a second from the time the eye sees light, it processes the information and sends it to the brain.

Camera Lens

The small black center of our eye is called a **pupil**. The **pupil draws in light** energy and then **transfers** that energy to our **brain** by way of the retina. The human eye works very much like a **camera** – the pupil of the eye and the shutter of a camera each control how much light is received. The **retina of the eye and the film of a camera each receive images** that are taken in by the available light. The brain then evaluates the colors according to what the eye has seen. The brain's ability to sense and understand light, energy and matter is truly phenomenal and enables us to decipher the color we are actually seeing.

Color Blindness

Dichromatism (di-chro-ma-tism) is a condition in which a person has difficulty viewing two of the primary colors such as red and green, or blue and yellow. **This is sometimes referred to as partial color blindness.**

Color blindness is when a person is unable to **visually differentiate between certain shades of color. Color receptors (cones) in the eye's retina are sensitive to red, green and blue wavelengths.** When someone is color-blind, he or she is unable to distinguish the color's wavelength and therefore the color range becomes distorted. Color blindness is typically present at birth, but may also occur through eye damage or disease. Eight to 12 percent of men are color-blind, and on average, tend to experience color blindness more than women. **Complete color blindness** is when the eyes perceive all color in variations of gray.

RED has the **LONGEST** wavelength

GREEN has a **MEDIUM** wavelength

BLUE/VIOLET has the **SHORTEST** wavelength

Categories of Color Blindness

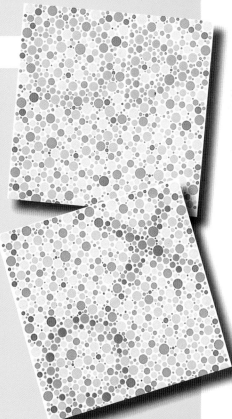

Protanopia (pro-ta-no-pi-a) **vision** is when an individual **cannot distinguish the color red** and at times, may confuse red with the color green. This is because the retina is devoid of red cone receptors.

Deuteranopia (deu-ter-a-no-pi-a) **vision** occurs when shades of **green are minimized or diminished.** The color red may also appear distorted along with shades of blue, violet and gray. The green cone receptors in the retina are missing or malfunctioning.

Tritanopia (tri-tan-o-pi-a) **vision mistakes blue for green colors and yellow for violet.** In this case, the blue cone receptors are absent in the retina of the eye. Tritanopia is a rare form of color deficiency generally affecting one out of 10,000 persons.

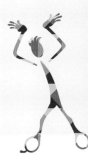

"In order to determine if you are color-blind and into which category of color blindness you fall ... schedule an appointment with an optometrist to get your vision checked and tested. For more information about taking a color vision test, refer to www.colorvisiontesting.com."

Natural Light ...

The colors we see when looking at an object are directly influenced by the **type and intensity of the light source** that hits the object. As haircolorists, we are taught that **natural light (daylight) is the ultimate source for determining a client's natural haircolor level.** While natural light is a good source in which to view true color, keep in mind that the color composition of natural light will change throughout the day.

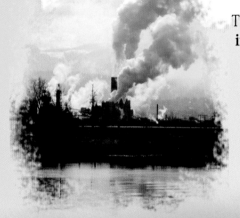

There are many **environmental and location factors that influence the color of the sky.** Pollutants, dust, weather, smog and location help determine a sky's color – even living near a volcano or in a big city will influence how the spectrum of colors are scattered. Remember, **natural sunlight** is derived from the spectrum of colors ranging from blue to violet. As a result, **each part of the day will vary in its color reflection.**

Dawn

As the sun begins to climb and light up the horizon (the sun is not in view yet), we will see **cool opalescent colors** in the sky. The clouds appear like iridescent pearl.

Sunrise

As the sun is rising above the horizon, the colors emitted are typically **yellows and oranges**, but depending on air clarity, pinks, grays or cool colors may be more evident.

Early Morning

The early morning light typically produces **cool tones with some gray** and by mid-morning the sky may turn to a silver or pastel yellow color.

Natural Light ...

Early Afternoon (Day)
Early afternoon brings **rich, true colors**.
The best part of the day to view color is from
mid-morning to mid-afternoon.

Late Afternoon
As the sun starts to descend in the late afternoon
sky, **cool tones are revealed through pastel
blues,** which then change over to more **vivid,
gold** colors. Painters and photographers prefer
this type of sunlight, because it **maximizes the
brilliance and beauty** of their artistic creations.

Sunset
As the sun descends from the sky,
the glow of **yellow changes to a
bright orange** and finishes with a
fiery ball of red, which spreads
across the horizon.

Dusk
Once the sun disappears from view, the sky
displays colors of **violet and dark blues.**

*"All of these various light changes will affect our perception of color.
Natural light is still your best source for viewing haircolor."*

Lighting Up Color ..

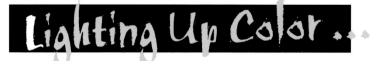

The types of lighting in a beauty salon and colors used to decorate the salon have an **impact when determining a client/guest's haircolor,** whether it is natural or artificial. When viewing completed haircoloring services, keep in mind **certain light sources have a negative impact** by producing unflattering results.

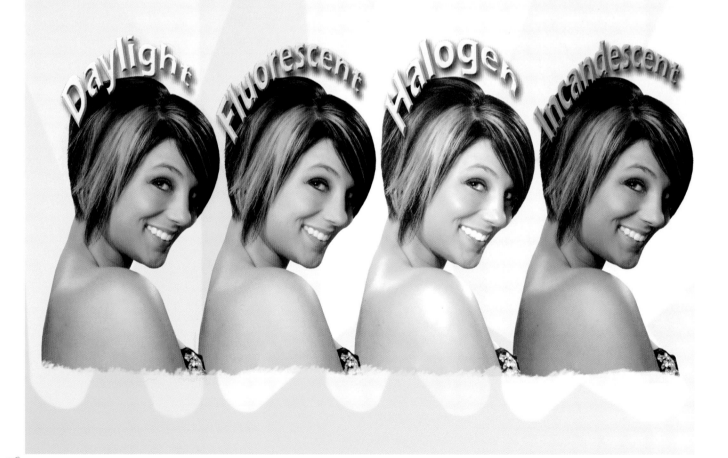

Daylight — Reflects true color

Fluorescent — Reflects cool/ash tones

Halogen — Reflects white/bright colors

Incandescent — Reflects warm/red colors

Daylight Fluorescent Halogen Incandescent

Lighting Up Color ...

Indoor Lighting Sources

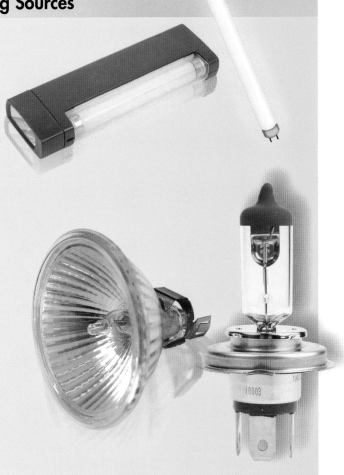

Fluorescent (fluo-res-cent) **lighting** is produced by a phosphor-coated glass tube filled with inert gas and mercury.

- Produces **cool to drab tones** on skin and hair, which can sometimes **appear green**
- Is the least expensive light source for the hair salon
- Is improved and comes in a variety of colors, types and sizes

Halogen (hal-o-gen) **lighting** comes from a more efficient version of the incandescent bulb and will last longer.

- Produces **crisp, bright, white light that is slightly warmer** in color than incandescent
- Maintains long-lasting light without fading
- Is a popular choice for use in a hair salon

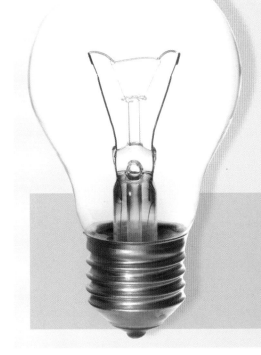

Incandescent (in-can-des-cent) **lighting** results from heating a metallic filament – usually made of the element **tungsten** (tung-sten), which is held inside a traditional glass light bulb.

- Provides soft effect that is suitable to face and hair
- Provides more heat than light
- Produces **warm to red (gold) tones**
- Is an expensive light source for use in a salon

The **Energy Independence and Security Act of 2007** mandates 25 percent greater efficiency for light bulbs, to be phased in from 2012 through 2014. Most incandescent light bulbs are slowly being removed from the U.S. market. Go to http://energy.senate.gov/public/_files/RL342941.pdf

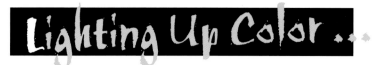

Cost Efficient Indoor Lighting Sources

Compact Fluorescent (fluo-res-cent) lighting or **CFL** is a newer version of fluorescent lighting that **uses less energy.** CFL lighting is created when an electric current passes over mercury, which then changes it to ultraviolet light. This UV light then passes over a phosphor-coating, converting it to visible light, all within a glass housing. The initial cost for this type of fluorescent lighting is higher than other kinds, but due to its long-term durability, money will be saved.

- Produces **less heat**
- Uses less energy, **long-lasting**
- High purchase cost, but efficient for long-term use

CAUTION: Follow "Go Green" safety tips for the handling and disposing of any broken fluorescent light bulbs, especially CFL bulbs due to their mercury content.
Go to www.recycleabulb.com.

Lighting Up Color ...

Light-Emitting Diode (di-ode) **or LED lighting** is the **modern technology for lighting** up a room/salon. This type of light source contains **no filament or mercury** – it uses a semi-conductor that produces light as the electricity goes through it.

- Energy efficient – long lifespan and lightweight
- Clean and powerful lighting
- Full spectrum lighting

NOTE: Diode is a device that converts alternating current to direct current.

"LED lighting is the most expensive, but requires less energy and is considered the best source of lighting for inside the salon. Although cheaper is not always better – sunlight is free and is the ideal light source for viewing color."

Color and Emotions

Emotions are an **individual's feelings** about something or someone. **Feelings** can range from happy to sad or peaceful to stressful or any other **type of expression.** A person's **surroundings can be influential** in the way he or she feels, whether it is positive or negative.

Light and color have a powerful effect on our perceptions and emotions. Human behavior and our reactions when viewing color and light have been studied and documented in various testing observations.

The brain is the largest mass of nerve tissue in the body; it is considered the "control center" for the nervous system. The cerebrum part of the brain is separated into four lobes with each one influencing certain functions. The brain regulates movement, sensation and the capability to think.

Frontal Lobe:
behavior, problem solving, initiative, eye movements, muscle movements, sense of smell, creative thoughts, reflections, intellect, attention

Parietal Lobe:
some reading, visual and language functions, sense of touch, responds to internal stimuli

Temporal Lobe:
fear, music, visual and auditory memory, some language, speech hearing and behavior functions, sense of identity

Occipital Lobe:
reading, vision

Color Therapy

Wherever color is placed and seen, it will have an effect on a person's behavior and emotions. The color of clothing worn, the application of makeup, color of the walls, furniture and flooring in a room also have an influence on a person's mood.

Color therapy is a natural therapeutic approach that **uses color to affect our emotions, moods and perhaps even our health.** When color is reflected back to the individual, the mood or emotion of that particular color is created, which can result in a personality change whether it is positive or negative.

The guide on this page shows some common reactions to haircolors. Keep in mind that haircolor not only affects the individual wearing it, but also everyone with whom that person interacts. These examples demonstrate the powerful effects of color – both positive and negative.

1

BLONDE

playful, positive, happy, talkative, wise, hyperactive, memorable, energetic

2

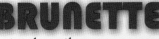

BRUNETTE

natural, earthy, reliable, genuine

RED

3

intense, passionate, fiery, exciting, angry, impatient, courageous, self-confident

BLACK

aloof, dominant, powerful, sophisticated

Surrounding Color ...

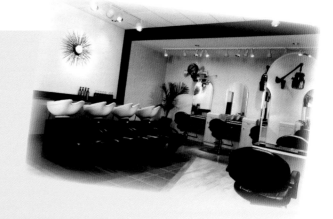

The wall colors in your haircoloring room will reflect on the client/guest's face and hair, so it is important to avoid strong or conflicting colors in that area. The optimum color choice to use would be a combination of the achromatic colors – **black and white.**

The **pure white room will reflect** all the colors of the spectrum, but creates a cold atmosphere. The **pure black room will absorb** all the colors of the spectrum and create a depressing environment. The best solution is a complementary mixture of both black and white.

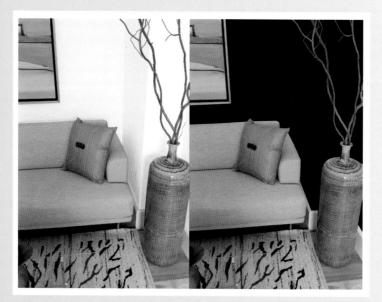

The following are a few examples of our psychological reactions to light and color, and the ways in which our mind sometimes plays tricks on us.

- People working in a room painted red, felt hot, while people working in another room painted blue, felt cool ... yet both of the room temperatures were 70 degrees.

- Prisoners locked in a red room felt angry, while other prisoners locked in a pink room felt calm, regardless of both rooms having the same size and dimension.

- A group of men and women lifted some objects in a black color, and then lifted those same size objects in a white color ... the black objects felt heavier.

Surrounding Color ...

There are many ways in which color can be related to other areas of life. Let us look at music and compare the haircolorist to the musical composer.

For example, some of the terminology used to describe the areas of a composer's work is similar to a haircolorist ... think of the words tone and harmony.

Tone for the composer means a distinct sound and for the colorist, it is the distinction of a color shade.

Harmony for the haircolorist is the synchronization of the elements of color with the overall design, and for the musical artist, it is a pleasing combination of sounds or notes that are sung together.

In addition, light has seven different colors (chromatic colors) – **red**, **orange**, **yellow**, **green**, **blue**, **indigo and violet** and musical scales have seven different notes – Do-Re-Mi-Fa-So-La-Ti. Just like a composer has unlimited creative potential using the combination of the seven notes in a scale, the haircolorist also has unlimited creative potential through the combination of the seven chromatic colors.

Musical notes are joined together to make beautiful melodies for **us to hear**, and **light** along with its **energy** will create the colors from the **visible light spectrum** for us to see.

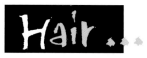
Hair *is a group of* **"thread-like"** *strands growing out from the skin or scalp. Hair is our medium upon which we create our art. It is our means for providing regular hair-care maintenance, chemical services and/or creative expression, and in the process, enhance a person's beauty. The technical term for the study of hair, disorders, diseases and hair-care is* **trichology** *(tri-kah-lu-gee).*

"For beautiful looking hair, eat healthy, exercise and keep hair and scalp clean."

Hair Shaft ...

The portion of hair that extends beyond the skin or scalp is the **hair shaft**.

The hair shaft consists of three layers:

Cuticle is the tough, outer protective covering. This layer is generally made of seven to **12 layers of transparent, overlapping scale-like (flat) cells**. Temporary haircolors coat the cuticle and semi-permanent haircolors penetrate.

Cortex is the soft, elastic, thick, inner layer made up of **elongated cells** that bond together tightly. This fibrous layer is **elastic (will stretch)**, and contains the **coloring matter (melanin)** and the hair's protein (keratin). The cortex is responsible for an estimated 90 percent of the hair's weight. Demi-permanent and permanent haircolor must enter the cortex in order for proper color development.

Medulla is the deepest layer, consisting of **round cells**. Sometimes it is intermittent or totally absent and is known to not have any true effect on the hair. Haircolor does not reach this layer.

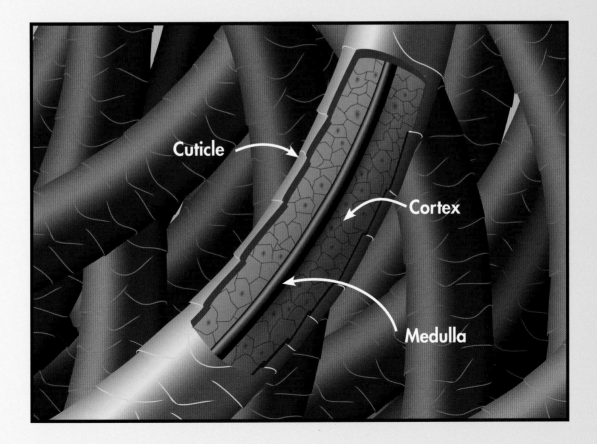

Cuticle

Cortex

Medulla

Hair Root ...

The portion of hair below the skin or scalp is **hair root.**

The hair root consists of the following structures:

Follicle (fol-li-cle) is the depression or pocket **surrounding the hair root.** Hair formation begins with the epidermis of skin or scalp, shifting downward into the dermis, which forms a channel and becomes the follicle. The **shape and direction of the follicle** determine the angle at which the hair fiber will emerge from the scalp.

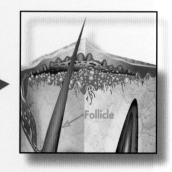

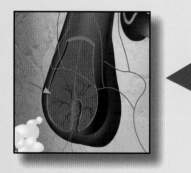

Bulb is the rounded club-shaped part at the **very end of the hair root.** It is hollowed out and fits over the dermal papilla. The bulb will come along with the hair when pulled from the scalp.

Dermal papilla (pa-pil-la) is a mass of tiny capillaries (blood) and nerves located directly **under the hollowed area of the hair bulb.** The dermal papilla **supplies oxygen and nourishment** for the continued growth of the hair fiber.

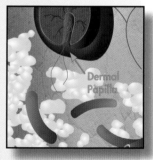

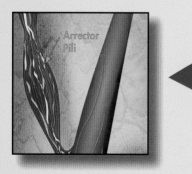

Arrector pili (a-rrec-tor pi-li) **muscle** is a small involuntary muscle located along the **side of the hair follicle.** This muscle is responsible for the **"goose flesh" or "goose bump"** appearance on the skin, which allows the hair to lift in a standing position due to a reaction from cold or fear.

Sebaceous (se-ba-ceous) glands are **"oil" glands** that produce the **oily substance called sebum.** Sebum acts as a lubricant (mixture of fats or lipids) for the hair as well as the skin and scalp. These glands appear as sacs that attach to the **upper sides of the hair follicle.**

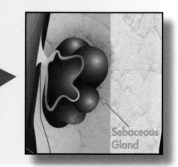

Hair Root ...

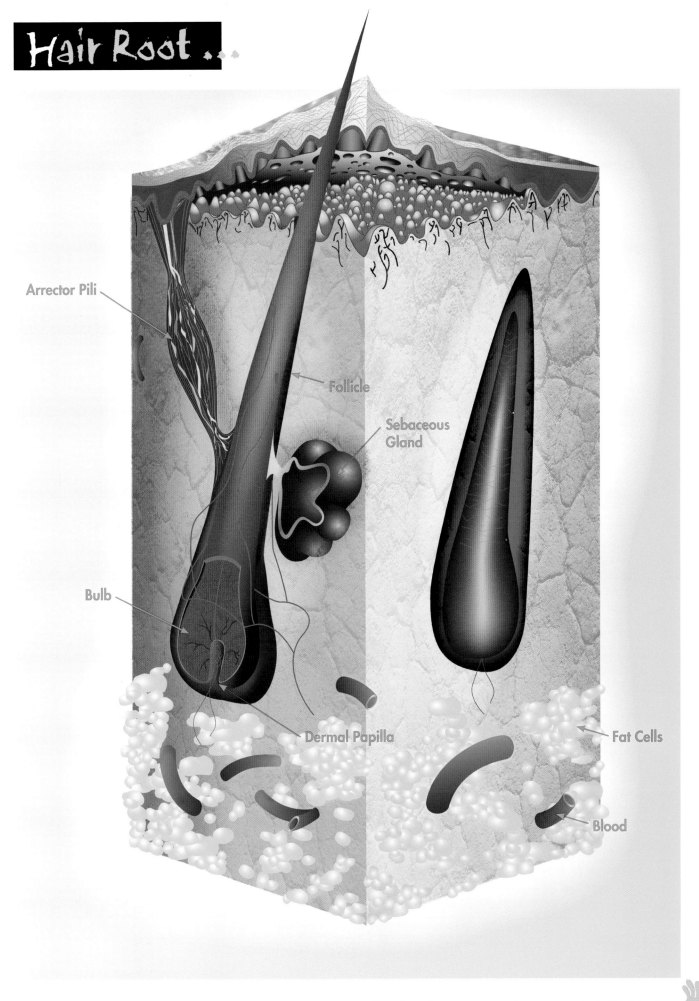

Arrector Pili

Follicle

Sebaceous
Gland

Bulb

Dermal Papilla

Fat Cells

Blood

As cosmetologists, we need to understand the composition of the hair in order to deliver **a competent and successful hair service.** *When performing chemical services, the knowledge of how the hair will possibly react to the chemical product* **provides confidence for the professional and trust from the client.**

The hair begins to form in the underlying layers (dermis) of the skin. Living cells collect in a pocket of skin located in the dermis layer, which starts the **process of building the hair root**. This pocket is referred to as the follicle. The **follicle** surrounds the entire root, providing a space or channel through which the hair root will emerge from the skin and scalp to become the hair shaft. These cells begin by moving upward inside the follicle, first maturing and **keratinizing (hardening)**, then dying and starting to form the structure (root) of the hair. As this process progresses, the hair continues to develop and gradually move out of the scalp creating the **hair shaft, a non-living fiber**.

Hair Shaft

Follicle

Hair Root

Bulb

"The only way to see inside the hair is with a powerful electron microscope."

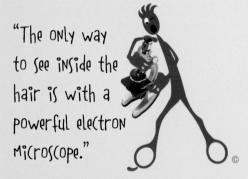

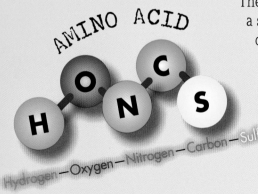

AMINO ACID

Hydrogen—Oxygen—Nitrogen—Carbon—Sulfur

The living cells that start this whole process are composed of a **strong, fibrous protein called keratin**. The protein is derived from the amino acids that make up the hair. The amino acids link together to form minute protein fibers. Each amino acid consists of the five elements, **6% hydrogen, 21% oxygen, 17% nitrogen, 51% carbon and 5% sulfur** ... an easier way of remembering is **HONCS!** These elements play an important role in the chemical breakdown for haircoloring and hair lightening.

Amino acids are connected by an **end bond or peptide bond** to form long, single chains referred to as a **polypeptide** or an **alpha helix coil.**

Three alpha helix coils twist around each other to form a **protofibril.**

Nine protofibrils are packaged together as a **bundle.**

Eleven bundles will produce a **microfibril.**

Hundreds of microfibrils are cemented together in a **fibrous protein bundle** referred to as a **macrofibril.**

This process continues with **hundreds of macrofibrils** grouped together to create a **cortical fiber.**

The **cortical fibers** are grouped together to produce the **cortex.** The dried, dead cells that surround the cortex are the **cuticle scales.**

Development of a single strand of hair:

Amino acids
Peptide bonds
Polypeptide chains (3)
Protofibrils (9)
Microfibrils (11)
Macrofibrils
Cortical fibers
Cuticle scales

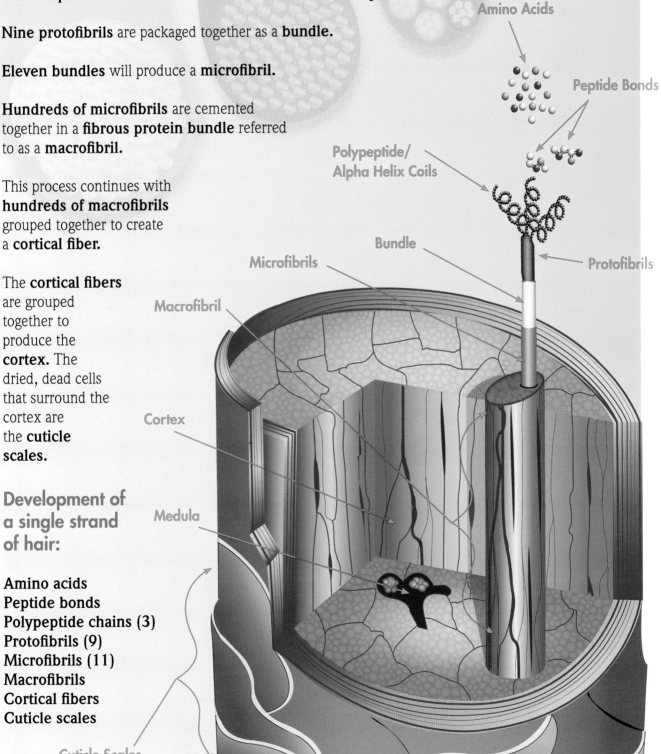

Amino Acids

Peptide Bonds

Polypeptide/
Alpha Helix Coils

Bundle

Protofibrils

Microfibrils

Macrofibril

Cortex

Medula

Cuticle Scales

Natural Color of Hair . . .

The natural color of our hair is derived from **melanocyte** (mel-a-no-cyte) **cells** that consist of a membrane body of **melanosomes**, which contain melanin (mel-a-nin). *Tyrosine* (ty-ro-sine) *is the* **amino acid** *found in the melanocyte cell. These cells are located in the* **cortex of the hair** *as well as in your skin and eyes.* **Melanin is the coloring matter** *that provides natural color to our hair and skin.*

The formula for naturally occurring melanin is:

+   **Tyrosine** (amino acid)
       Enzymes (biochemical catalyst)

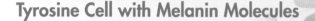

=   Molecules of Eumelanin and Pheomelanin

Tyrosine Cell with Melanin Molecules

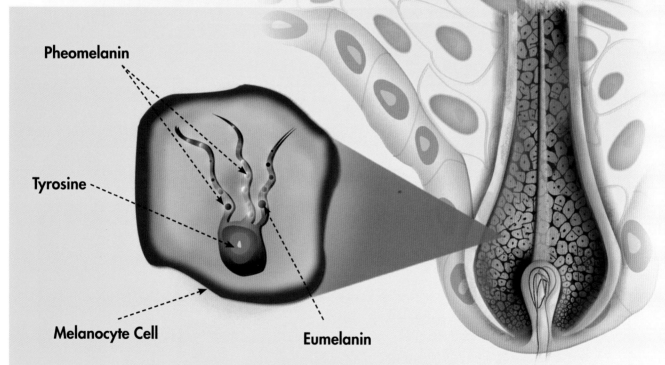

Pheomelanin

Tyrosine

Melanocyte Cell

Eumelanin

There are three types of melanin:

Eumelanin (eu-mel-a-nin) produces **brown** to **black** pigments in the hair.

Pheomelanin (phe-o-mel-a-nin) produces **yellow** to **red** pigments in the hair.

Mixed melanin is a combination of eumelanin and pheomelanin inside one melanocyte cell.

Natural Color of Hair ...

Natural haircolors will vary in appearance with each individual depending on ratio of eumelanin to pheomelanin, concentration of pigment (density of color), hereditary and environmental factors.

Dark hair has a **high eumelanin production** and concentration of pigment/melanin, whether it is a dark brown or dark blonde.

1

Gray hair occurs with a **gradual or slowing down of melanin** production in the cortex of the hair. This hair still has some melanin in order to produce the gray appearance, but the concentration of pigment is slowly decreasing from the hair.

Blonde hair has a **low concentration** of both types of melanin – specifically **eumelanin**. A slight amount of **pheomelanin** exists to provide the color of yellow for the blonde hair.

White hair has a **total absence of pigment – no eumelanin or pheomelanin**. Typically as the human body ages (depending on each individual), the hair will slowly progress from pigmented hair to no pigment or white hair.

When melanin begins to **naturally decrease in concentration,** *the haircolor will be altered to reflect this change. Gray hair is a decline in the production of melanin, resulting in low amounts of eumelanin and pheomelanin, which creates varying concentrations of remaining pigments.*

Gray hair appears as having a **combination of white and pigmented hair** (ringed hair), with the pigmented hair eventually fading to white. The decrease in melanin production occurs during the catagen and telogen life cycle of hair growth, which explains the slow progression of all the hair turning to white. The medical term for **gray hair is canities** (can-nish-eez).

Canities

Gray Hair ...

The two types of canities are:

Acquired canities is when the melanocytes gradually become inactive and **production of melanin is slowed** down turning hair to a gray color that varies in pigment concentration. This typically occurs as the human body ages and/or genetics.

Congenital canities can occur before or at birth. **Albinism** is the best example of melanin production slowing down or being totally absent. An **albino** is genetically afflicted with no coloring matter over his or her entire body.

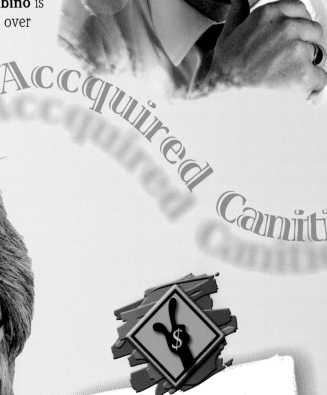

Accquired Canities

Introducing the benefits of haircoloring services to client/guests with gray hair will help them feel and look young again as well as keep them coming back to the salon for color maintenance!

The distribution *of natural melanin in the hair varies according to texture, therefore processing times and shades of color achieved will also vary according to texture.*

Texture is the measurement and/or tactile quality of each hair fiber's diameter.

Diameter refers to the thickness or width of a single strand of hair.

The following is an overview of the three basic hair fiber textures/diameters and their reactions to haircoloring and hair lightening.

Three Types of Hair Textures/Diameters are:

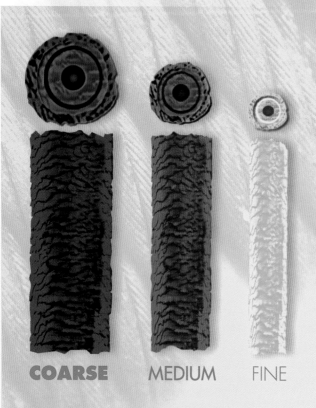

COARSE   MEDIUM   FINE

Coarse hair has a **large diameter/width** and feels thick. The color pigments are spread out within the cortex due to the hair strand width. This may create some resistance in the haircoloring and hair lightening process.

Medium hair has an **average diameter/thickness** and is used as a baseline for both processing time and accuracy of color achieved.

Fine hair has a **small diameter/width** and feels thin. The color pigments are grouped close together in the cortex of the hair. This may create a fast development time when processing haircolor and/or hair lightener.

The texture of hair is also described as the **tactile quality or feel of the hair surface.** This is generally influenced by the natural tempo or movement within the hair strand, which is determined by the shape of the hair follicle. The structure of hair can be **naturally straight, wavy or curly.**

Hair Texture ...

Three Hair Follicle Shapes are:

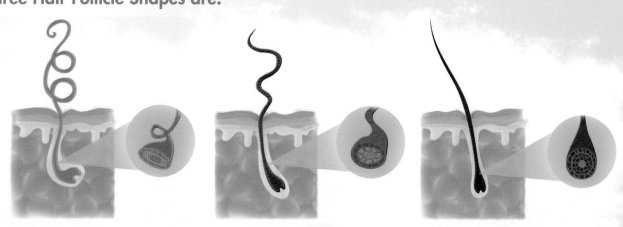

1. **Narrow Oval or Flat-shaped follicle** produces **curly** hair.

2. **Large Oval follicle** produces **wavy** hair.

3. **Round or Circular follicle** produces **straight** hair.

The surface of the hair is typically influenced by the condition of the cuticle layer, which is related to the porosity of the hair. If the cuticle scales are raised, the hair will not have a smooth texture, but instead feel rough to the touch. If the cuticle scales are lying flat, the hair surface will feel smooth.

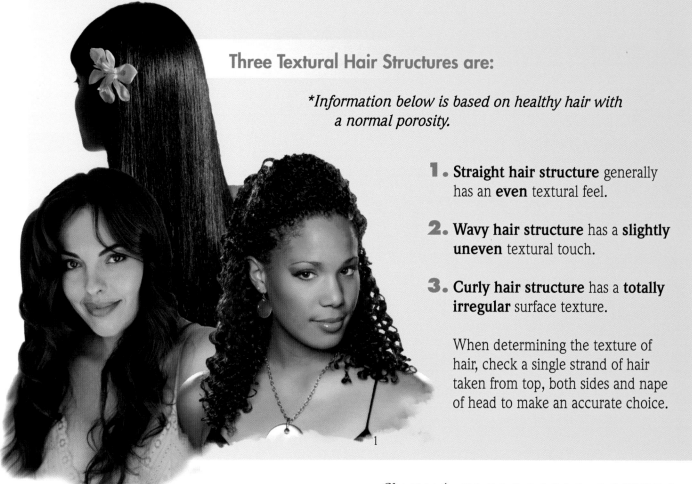

Three Textural Hair Structures are:

*Information below is based on healthy hair with a normal porosity.

1. **Straight hair structure** generally has an **even** textural feel.

2. **Wavy hair structure** has a **slightly uneven** textural touch.

3. **Curly hair structure** has a **totally irregular** surface texture.

When determining the texture of hair, check a single strand of hair taken from top, both sides and nape of head to make an accurate choice.

1

Hair Density ...

Take both hands and run them through your hair (or client/guest's hair) along the scalp – does it feel like you have a lot of hair on your head? Make sure you are checking the amount of hair on the head, as opposed to evaluating individual hair strands (texture of hair).

Three Types of Density are:

Density is the number of hair strands per square inch (2.5 cm) on the scalp. The average number of hair strands on the scalp is 100,000. This may vary depending upon natural haircolor, heredity, medication or hair-care.

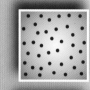

Thin density has **few** hair strands per square inch on the scalp.

Medium density has an **average** amount of hair strands per square inch on the scalp.

Thick density has the **most hair** strands per square inch on the scalp.

When evaluating density, consider the distribution of hair on all areas of the head. Some locations of the head, such as the hairline, crown and nape areas, may have a thin amount of hair with the remaining locations being thicker in density.

Natural Haircolor	Amount of Hair on Head
Blonde	140,000
Brown	110,000
Black	108,000
Red	80,000

When analyzing for density, part hair with comb and check the crown, hairline, both sides and nape of head.

Hair Density

Texture and density are sometimes misinterpreted as having the same meaning, but texture is analyzed by using a single strand of hair whereas density is determined by analyzing all the hair on the head. Keep in mind, a client/guest with coarse texture hair may have a thin hair density or a person with fine texture hair might have a thick hair density. Both texture and density need to be evaluated separately.

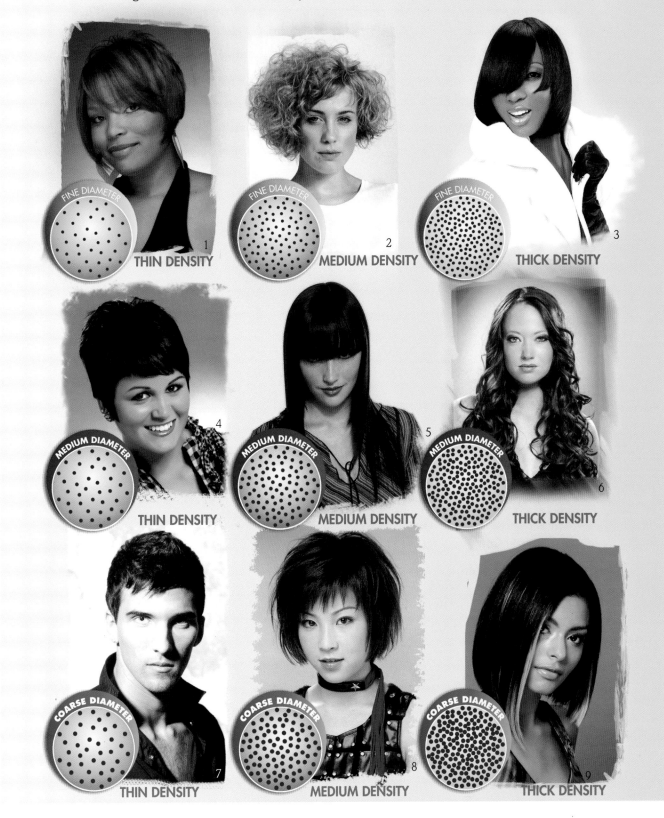

FINE DIAMETER
THIN DENSITY 1

FINE DIAMETER
MEDIUM DENSITY 2

FINE DIAMETER
THICK DENSITY 3

MEDIUM DIAMETER
THIN DENSITY 4

MEDIUM DIAMETER
MEDIUM DENSITY 5

MEDIUM DIAMETER
THICK DENSITY 6

COARSE DIAMETER
THIN DENSITY 7

COARSE DIAMETER
MEDIUM DENSITY 8

COARSE DIAMETER
THICK DENSITY 9

Hair Porosity ...

The penetration and development time *of haircolor and hair lightening is* **greatly influenced by the condition of the hair; the cuticle layer.** *The amount of water/liquid the hair (cuticle) absorbs within a relative amount of time is referred to as* **porosity** *(po-ros-i-ty). Much like a sponge, the hair will absorb water, but how long does the hair take to get wet? This is mostly determined by the condition of the cuticle. The* **cuticle is constructed of scales** *and if these scales are abraded or lifted, the hair will absorb liquids a lot quicker than hair that has cuticle scales lying flat.*

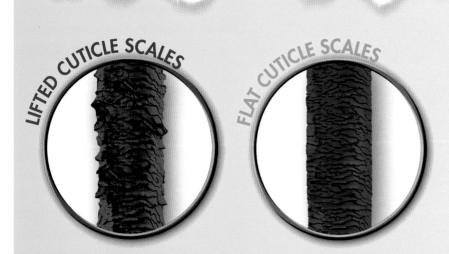

LIFTED CUTICLE SCALES   FLAT CUTICLE SCALES

Hair that has been improperly maintained or treated with any type of chemicals will have the cuticle scales raised to a certain degree. The depth of the lifted scales will be a factor in water absorption.

Four Types of Porosity are:

Resistant porosity has the **cuticle scales lying flat**, making the amount of liquid absorbed minimal.

Normal porosity has an average amount of absorption, considering the hair is in **"good condition."** This hair is usually maintained properly by using professional pH hair-care products.

Severe porosity is when the **cuticle scales are raised** due to damage by either chemical services or use of harsh hair-care tools.

Irregular porosity is usually indicated by the **combination of severe porosity** on the ends with **resistant or normal porosity** on the mid-strand. This can be due to heavy use of heating tools, improper chemical services and/or irregular haircut visits.

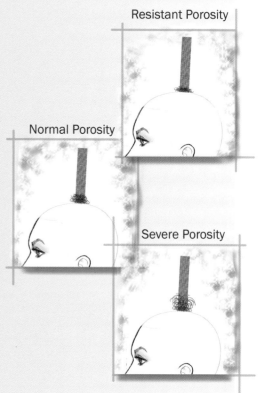

Resistant Porosity

Normal Porosity

Severe Porosity

Hair Porosity

ACTIVITY

Pair students together to perform the finger slide test and the water test on each other following the step-by-step procedures listed below to determine porosity of hair.

Finger Slide Test

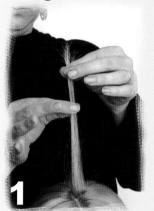

1
When checking for type of porosity, take a **small subsection of hair at top of head.** Both sides of head and nape area should be checked.

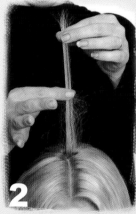

2
Slide fingers down hair shaft, similar to backcombing, till a cushioning of hair appears.

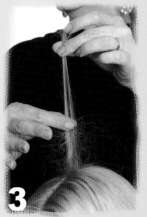

3
The **amount of hair pushed down to scalp** area will determine the type of porosity. If a lot of hair cushions at the scalp, cuticle scales are raised. If minimal amount of hair cushions at scalp, cuticle scales are compact.

Water Test

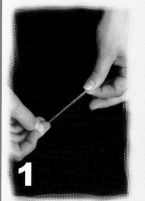

1
Cut a small subsection of hair from an inconspicuous area of the head (preferably near nape area).

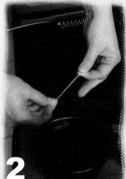

2
Hold subsection of hair with both hands at hair ends.

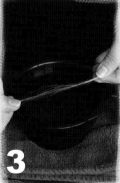

3
Grip hair ends tightly.

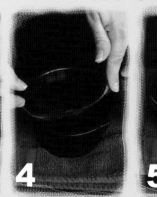

4
Place hair into water – watch hair become saturated.

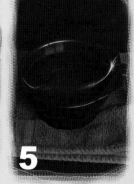

5
Hair is absorbing water inside bowl. If hair absorbs water quickly, cuticle scales are raised. If hair becomes saturated with water slowly, cuticle scales are lying flat.

Hair Elasticity

Why is hair able to endure lots of pulling and tugging through combing, brushing, etc. and yet still remain on the head? This is because the **hair is elastic**, which means it is able to stretch and return to its original length. **Elasticity** (e-las-tic-i-ty) is the capability of the hair strand to stretch and return to its previous form without breaking. The **twisted fibrils in the structure of the cortex** supply strength to the hair, resulting in haircolor longevity.

Two Types of Elasticity are:

1. **Average elasticity** on **wet hair** generally can be stretched **50 percent of its length** or if hair is **dry, usually 1/5 its length.**

2. **Low elasticity** hair will **break easily** due to the use of harsh hair-care products or being chemically overprocessed.

When analyzing for elasticity, take a single strand of dry hair from top, both sides and nape of head and slightly pull hair. If hair stretches and returns to its shape, much like a rubber band, then it has average strength. If hair breaks or does not return to its original length, then elasticity is considered low.

ACTIVITY

Pair students together to perform the elasticity test on each other following the step-by-step procedures listed below to determine elasticity of hair.

Elasticity Testing on Wet Hair

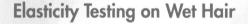

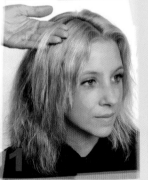
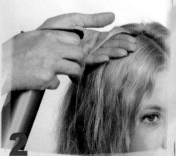
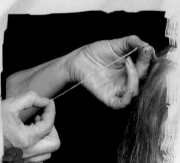
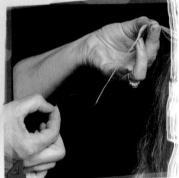

Select a **small subsection of hair** at top of head. Both sides of head and nape area should be checked.

Wet hair with water bottle – entire subsection must be wet.

With one hand, **hold subsection of hair** near scalp and with opposite hand, hold hair ends.

Slightly pull on subsection of hair, checking if hair breaks or will return to original shape once released from fingers. *This image shows some hair breakage.*

Hair Growth ...

Hair has the unique ability to grow, thereby creating varying lengths and multiple hairstyles in which to accommodate each person's creative image. Much like in nature, our **hair grows in stages or life cycle phases** and is greatly affected by our health and emotional well-being. At varying rates or simultaneously, single strands of hair will grow and shed on an individual's head.

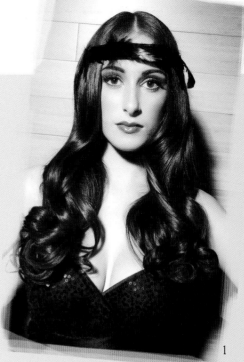

1

Three stages of hair growth:

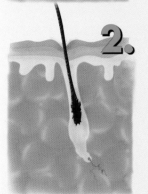

1. Anagen (an-a-gen) **or growing stage** is when the hair continues to survive and grow at an average **½ inch** (1.25 cm) **per month**, which depends upon each person and the location of hair. **Two to six years is the life expectancy** of hair in this stage, but may last as long as 10 years.

2. Catagen (cat-a-gen) **or intermediary** (in-ter-me-di-ar-y) **stage** is when the hair **stops growing** and begins the process of **disconnecting from the papilla and follicle.** The follicle channel gets smaller to about ⅓ (0.84 cm) its length, the hair bulb recedes and the withered hair root end becomes clubbed-shaped. Melanin production stops and the hair root changes to a white appearance. This process may **last two to three weeks.**

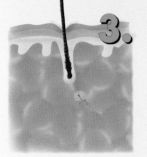

3. Telogen (tel-o-gen) **or shedding (or resting) stage** is when the **hair cycle ends** and the **hair rests** and eventually **sheds from the skin or scalp.** At the end of this **three to six month phase**, the anagen stage will resume with new hair growth in the same hair follicle from which the hair was shed. The hair might not shed in this stage, but be pushed out by new hair growth in the anagen stage.

All three stages repeat numerous times and in different sequences within the follicles; therefore, at any one point in time, we have an average of **90 percent hair on our heads.** The remaining **10 percent hair is in the telogen stage.**

Facts About Hair Growth

- Health can affect hair growth. Lack of vitamins/minerals, certain medications, illness or an injury to skin or scalp can all have an impact.

- **Normal daily hair loss** is an average of **30 to 50 hair strands**, which are then replaced by new hair.

- Hair grows on all areas of the body with the exception of the palms of hands, soles of feet, lips and eyelids.

- Weather affects hair loss, with more hair being shed during the cold months, while warm temperatures will activate the growing (anagen) stage of hair.

- Haircutting or shaving has **no effect** on the growth of hair because hair grows underneath the scalp beginning at the papilla.

- During a woman's menstrual cycle or pregnancy, hair does not grow faster. In fact, hair growth typically slows down while pregnant.

1

Action of Haircolor ...

*O*nce we understand *the ingredients that make up the artificial haircolor that we use on our hair, then we need to learn how that same* **color can alter or completely change our own natural haircolor.** *The possibilities are endless in changing a person's haircolor when using a wide variety of shades/colors available to us. In order to achieve this true phenomenon and have a successful haircolor service, the cosmetologist needs to understand how the color affects the hair, along with its delivery and development.*

1

Temporary, semi-permanent, demi-permanent and permanent haircolors each have a different effect on the hair. Each type of color varies according to what layer of hair the color develops, the strength of the haircolor and its durability. As explained in the science chapter, the color molecules for each of these haircolors range in size and strength, therefore affecting the color's penetration into the layers of hair.

2

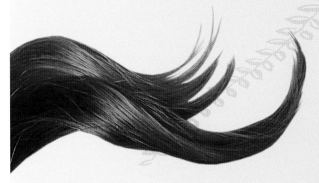

Temporary and semi-permanent haircolors are considered non-oxidative and contain direct dyes. Demi-permanent, permanent color and lighteners require hydrogen peroxide, which creates the chemical reaction called oxidation, in order to develop their color.

DISCLAIMER: *As a reminder, the information provided on these pages is a general overview of how each category of haircolor reacts to the hair. We highly recommend that you always read the manufacturer's instructions before handling any haircolor or hair lightener product.*

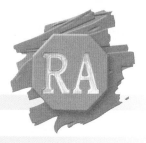

Non-Oxidative Haircolor (physical change):

Temporary haircolor coats the hair surface – covering ONLY the cuticle layer. This haircolor will **only last until the hair is shampooed**, which will depend on how often the hair is cleansed. The color molecules are large, so they cannot penetrate the cuticle layer unless hair porosity is other than normal. If cuticle scales are raised or a person's hair is light in color, the temporary color penetrates further into the cuticle layer and creates a color stain. This would result in a temporary color lasting beyond the first cleansing treatment, gradually fading from the hair with each shampoo. Temporary color creates a **physical change** to the hair, which can **ONLY add color or go darker.** Temporary color cannot create a lighter level of color than a person's natural level of haircolor.

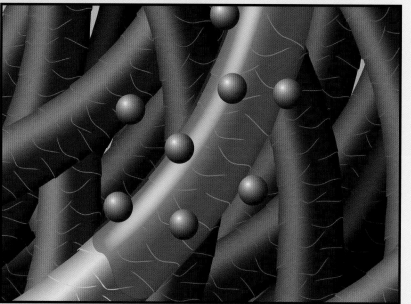

Advantages	Disadvantages
Provides haircolor without a permanent change	Color can wipe off and/or stain the skin and hair
Safe for use on most client/guests – generally NO patch test is required	Moisture and/or perspiration can cause color to stain the skin
Can use as a gentle toner on bleached hair	**Cannot** lighten hair – only **add color** to the existing haircolor
Helps to reduce the appearance of yellow undertones	May not have consistent (even) color coverage
Tones down white or gray hair	Color only remains in hair till next shampoo
A retouch service is not required	

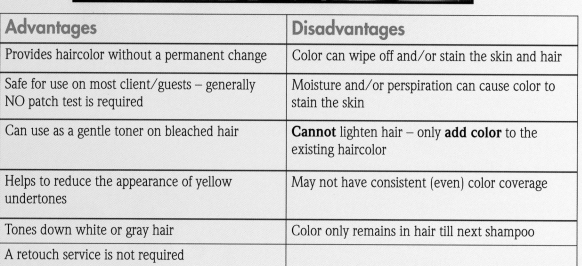

Place a retail display unit near your styling station to provide great product visibility and awareness. Encourage your client/guests to purchase color enhancing shampoos to brighten or tone their hair between salon visits.

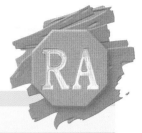

Non-Oxidative Haircolor (physical change):

Semi-permanent haircolor has the ability to **partially penetrate the cuticle layer** due to small color molecules. The direct dyes (color) from the bottle are placed on the hair – no other chemicals are added in the color mixture. The end color result is a combination of the client/guest's existing haircolor and the applied semi-permanent color. The semi-permanent color **DOES NOT reach the cortex** unless the porosity is less than normal. Porosity of hair has a great impact on color absorption, durability and color intensity. Semi-permanent color generally **lasts four to six shampoos** depending on how often the hair is cleansed. This type of color **gradually fades**; typically there is **no appearance of new growth**, which means retouching is usually not necessary.

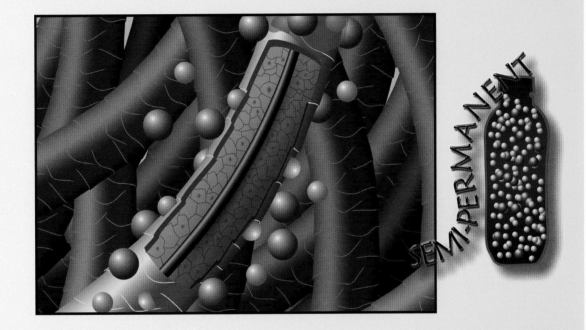

Advantages	Disadvantages
Color will not wipe off and/or stain the skin	Color inconsistencies due to color gradually fading
Color retouching (usually) not required – check with manufacturer	Color coverage for gray and white hair may be inconsistent
Provides haircolor without a permanent change – a good introductory color	Any heat intensity may increase fading of color
No H_2O_2 added – color is directly from bottle	**Cannot** lighten natural haircolor – only deposits color
	Lasts four to six shampoos

Action of Haircolor . . .

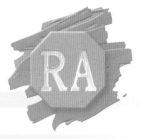

Oxidative Haircolor (chemical change):

Demi-permanent haircolor is an oxidative color that **does not contain ammonia,** but is mixed with a low volume of hydrogen peroxide or other type of oxidizer. Due to small color molecules and the addition of a low volume H_2O_2, the **color penetrates the cuticle and goes partially into the cortex.** Once these molecules enter the cortex, they link together, which locks them in place and enables the color to last longer. Demi-permanent color may **last four to six weeks** depending on how often hair is shampooed. The concentration of alkalizing agents in this less aggressive haircolor is minimal; however, due to the slight lifting of cuticle scales, the hair's pH must be restored and maintained at a 4.5 to 5.5 with the use of professional liquid tools. A **predisposition test is required 24 to 48 hours** prior to haircolor service to check if client/guest has sensitivity/allergy to the demi-permanent color.

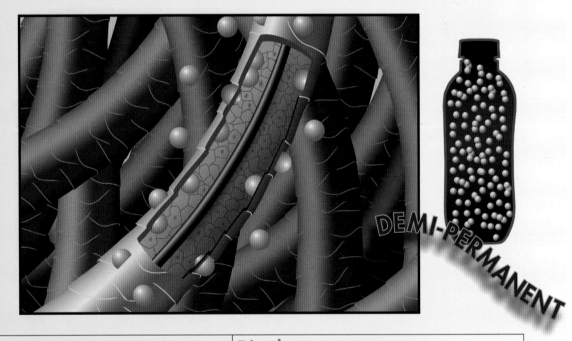

DEMI-PERMANENT

Advantages	Disadvantages
Provides haircolor without a permanent change – a good introductory color	Can ONLY go darker or deposit color, **NO lifting** of natural haircolor
Use as a refresher on existing haircolor	Requires a low volume hydrogen peroxide
Can cover or blend low percentages of gray hair	Predisposition test is required
Use for color correction	Slight fading of haircolor along with re-growth
Lasts four to six weeks	

"Remember, if hair porosity is other than normal, penetration of haircolor will be inconsistent."

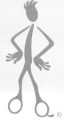

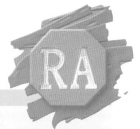

Action of Haircolor...

Oxidative Haircolor (chemical change):

Permanent haircolor is an oxidative color that **does contain ammonia or other types of alkalizing agents,** which are designed to be **mixed with varying volumes of hydrogen peroxide.** The beauty of permanent color is its ability to change a person's haircolor to almost any desired color, whether he or she wants light or dark colors or even a combination of both. This is accomplished by the small colorless molecules referred to as **aniline derivative colors** (an-i-line de-riv-a-tive), which are derived from coal tar dyes (synthetic).When these dyes are combined with hydrogen peroxide and an alkalizing agent such as ammonia or alkanolamines, they become larger and lock in place inside the cortex of the hair … hence the name "permanent." The **ammonia or alkalizing agent swells the cuticle layer, raising the scales,** which allows the dye intermediates to enter the cortex and alter the natural melanin. Permanent haircolor generally lasts **four to six weeks** until new growth appears, resulting in a retouch color application.

The **two types of dye intermediates** used in aniline derivative colors/permanent color are **paraphenylenediamine** (para-phe-ni-lene-i-dia-mine) and **paratoluenediamine** (para-tol-u-ene-dia-mine). A **predisposition test is required 24 to 48 hours** prior to the haircolor service to check if client/guest has sensitivity/allergy to the permanent color.

Oxidative haircolor cannot lighten or lift existing artificial pigments. A reputable manufacturer's color remover product is specifically designed to remove artificial pigment.

"Permanent color works hand-in-hand with depositing artificial color while at the same time, lightens the natural melanin in the hair."

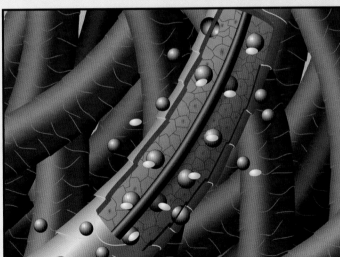

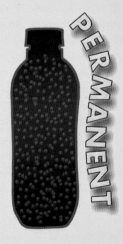

PERMANENT

Advantages	Disadvantages
Lasts four to six weeks	Patch test is required
Can go lighter and/or darker	Retouching is necessary
Create an endless variety of haircolors	May contain ammonia or other alkalizing agents – high pH
Excellent coverage of gray or white hair	High level colors have a tendency to fade/resistant to proper coverage

Action of Hair Lightener ...

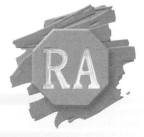

Oxidative (chemical change):

Hair lightener lifts the natural or artificial pigments from the cortex of the hair. In order for this to be accomplished, the lightener contains an alkaline agent such as alkanolamines or ammonia to **soften and swell the cuticle scales.** Hydrogen peroxide is then added to create the lightener mixture, which will increase the decolorization process through the H_2O_2 decomposition – called oxidation, or releasing of oxygen. The **melanin located in the cortex begins to scatter or diffuse,** resulting in a reflection of light color shades.

Lightener has a pH of 10 and is a strong alkalizing agent, which increases the chances for hair damage. Therefore it is very important to use professional hair-care products to restore hair to its normal pH.

Some haircolor procedures require the **application of a toner (haircolor product)** once lightener is removed from the hair. For this reason, a patch test is required 24 to 48 hours prior to haircolor service.

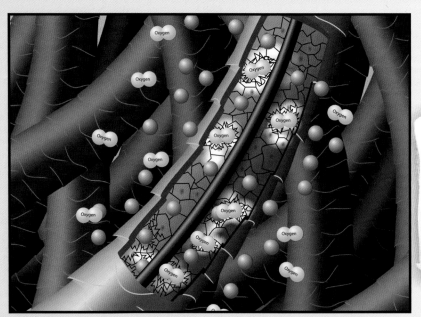

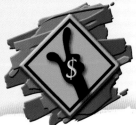

Market home maintenance hair-care products to the client/guest to restore hair back to a pH of 4.5 to 5.5.

Advantages	Disadvantages
Achieve light levels of color	Patch test is required because of toner application
Can create multiple fun and fashionable colors	High pH of 10 – contains alkalizing agents
No fading when using lightener	High maintenance – retouching is required
Lasts until appearance of new hair growth	Increase in hair damage/limit use of other chemicals such as permanent waves or chemical relaxers
Fast development time	

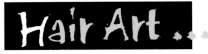

Hair Art ..

The biological powers *that define who we are also make each of us individuals with a unique combination of cultural and genetic traits and features. Each client/guest's hair is unique to that client/guest. As a professional haircolorist, you will use your knowledge and creativity to develop formulas that provide fabulous results to suit each of your clients/guests.*

THE CANVAS
Hair

THE ART MEDIUM
Haircolor

Not only is hair different in texture, it also differs in its natural haircolor and health of hair (porosity). Therefore, each new client/guest becomes a new canvas on which to color!

THE RESULTS
Different for each head of hair!

Light strikes an object and that object becomes

ILLUMINATED!

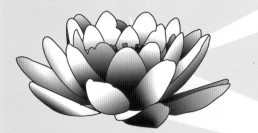

The **illuminated** object is captured by the human eye, processed and then transferred to our brains into a message.

This message is transformed, which allows us to experience the visual beauty of life that surrounds us every day!

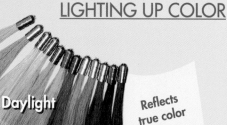

LIGHTING UP COLOR

The types of lighting in a beauty salon and colors used to decorate the salon have an **impact when determining a client/guest's haircolor,** whether it is natural or artificial. When viewing completed haircoloring services, keep in mind **certain light sources have a negative impact** by producing unflattering results.

Daylight	Reflects true color
Fluorescent	Reflects cool/ash tones
Halogen	Reflects white/bright colors
Incandescent	Reflects warm/red colors

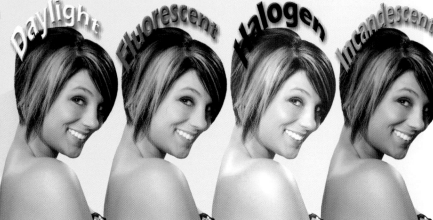

Daylight   Fluorescent   Halogen   Incandescent

Hair Shaft ...

THE HAIR SHAFT CONSISTS OF THREE LAYERS

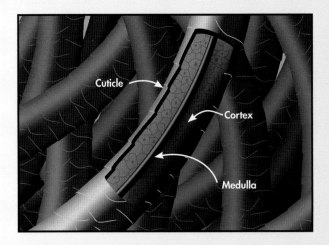

Cuticle is the tough, outer protective covering. This layer is generally made of seven to **12 layers of transparent, overlapping scale-like (flat) cells**. Temporary haircolors coat the cuticle and semi-permanent haircolors penetrate.

Cortex is the soft, elastic, thick, inner layer made up of **elongated cells** that bond together tightly. This fibrous layer is **elastic (will stretch)**, and contains the **coloring matter (melanin)** and the hair's **protein (keratin).** Demi-permanent and permanent haircolor must enter the cortex in order for proper color development.

Medulla is the deepest layer, consisting of **round cells**. Haircolor does not reach this layer.

NATURAL COLOR OF HAIR

The natural color of our hair is derived from **melanocyte** (mel-a-no-cyte) **cells** that consist of a membrane body of **melanosomes**, which contain **melanin**. These cells are located in the cortex of the hair as well as in your skin and eyes. **Melanin is the coloring matter** that provides natural color to our hair and skin.

THERE ARE THREE TYPES OF MELANIN

Eumelanin (eu-mel-a-nin) produces **brown** to **black** pigments in the hair.

Pheomelanin (phe-o-mel-a-nin) produces yellow to **red** pigments in the hair.

Mixed melanin is a combination of eumelanin and pheomelanin inside one melanocyte cell.

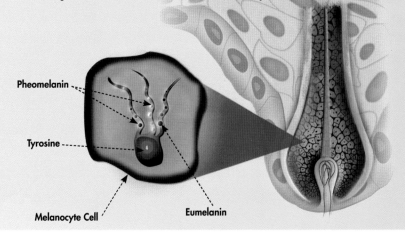

Action of Haircolor

NON-OXIDATIVE HAIRCOLOR (PHYSCIAL CHANGE):

Temporary haircolor coats the hair surface – covering ONLY the cuticle layer. This haircolor will **only last until the hair is shampooed**, which will depend on how often the hair is cleansed. The color molecules are large, so they can not penetrate the cuticle layer.

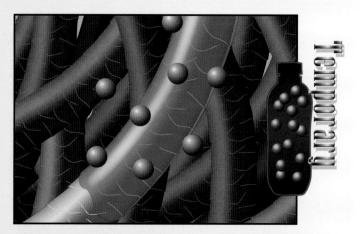

Semi-permanent haircolor has the ability to **partially penetrate the cuticle layer** due to small color molecules. The direct dyes (color) from the bottle are placed on the hair – no other chemicals are added in the color mixture. Semi-permanent color generally **lasts four to six shampoos** depending on how often the hair is cleansed. This type of color gradually fades.

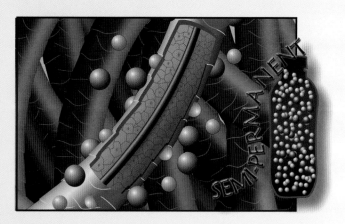

OXIDATIVE HAIRCOLOR (CHEMICAL CHANGE):

Demi-permanent haircolor is an oxidative color that **does not contain ammonia**, but is mixed with a low volume of hydrogen peroxide. Due to small color molecules and the addition of a low volume H_2O_2, the **color penetrates the cuticle and goes partially into the cortex**. Demi-permanent color may **last four to six weeks** depending on how often hair is shampooed.

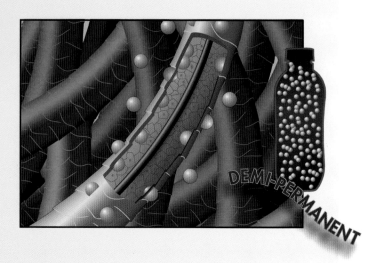

OXIDATIVE HAIRCOLOR (CHEMICAL CHANGE):

Permanent haircolor is an oxidative color that **does contain ammonia or other types of alkalizing agents,** which are designed to be **mixed with varying volumes of hydrogen peroxide.** This is accomplished by the small colorless molecules referred to as **aniline derivative colors** (an-i-line de-riv-a-tive), which are derived from coal tar dyes (synthetic). Permanent haircolor generally lasts **four to six weeks** until new growth appears at the scalp.

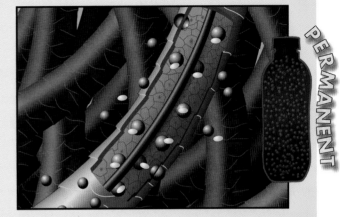

PERMANENT

ACTION OF HAIR LIGHTENER

Hair Lightener lifts the natural or artificial pigments from the cortex of the hair. In order for this to be accomplished, the lightener contains an alkaline agent such as alkanolamines or ammonia to **soften and swell the cuticle scales.** Hydrogen peroxide is then added to create the lightener mixture. The **melanin located in the cortex begins to scatter or diffuse,** resulting in a reflection of light color shades.

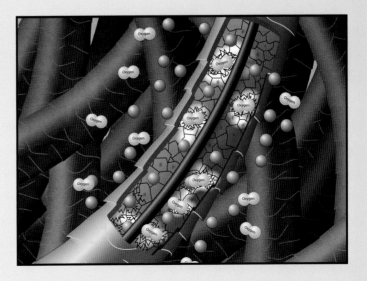

MULTIPLE CHOICE

1. Which layer of the hair contains melanin?
   A. cuticle   B. cortex   C. medulla

2. Which light source brings cool to drab tones to the skin and hair?
   A. incandescent   B. halogen   C. fluorescent

3. How long does permanent haircolor last?
   A. until hair is shampooed   B. four to six shampoos   C. four to six weeks

4. What category of color-blind vision cannot distinguish the color red?
   A. protanopia   B. deuteranopia   C. tritanopia

5. What is the strong fibrous protein that makes up the hair?
   A. keratin   B. melanin   C. enzyme

6. What happens to the melanin when a lightener is applied to the hair?
   A. increases   B. diffuses   C. hardens

7. What layer of the hair accepts semi-permanent color?
   A. cuticle   B. cortex   C. medulla

8. Which haircolor can lighten the natural melanin?
   A. semi-permanent   B. demi-permanent   C. permanent

9. Which type of melanin produces yellow to red pigments in the hair?
   A. eumelanin   B. pheomelanin   C. keratin

10. The natural haircolor associated with a **larger amount** of hair on the head is?
    A. blonde   B. brown   C. red

11. Which hair analysis area affects haircolor penetration and development time?
    A. density   B. porosity   C. elasticity

12. Which type of haircolor creates the chemical reaction called oxidation?
    A. semi-permanent   B. demi-permanent   C. temporary

13. What area of the hair root supplies nourishment for continued hair fiber growth?
    A. follicle   B. bulb   C. dermal papilla

14. Which type of haircolor contains ammonia?
    A. permanent   B. temporary   C. semi-permanent

15. Which type of haircolor penetrates the cuticle and partially into the cortex?
    A. temporary   B. semi-permanent   C. demi-permanent

16. What test is done 24 to 48 hours prior to the haircolor service to check for client/guest sensitivity to product?
    A. patch   B. strand   C. porosity

17. Which type of haircolor needs NO retouching?
    A. temporary   B. permanent   C. lightener

18. Name the hair growth stage when the hair cycle ends and the hair rests?
    A. anagen   B. catagen   C. telogen

19. What shape follicle produces wavy hair?
    A. round   B. large oval   C. narrow oval

20. What is the average growth of hair per month?
    A. 1 inch (2.5 cm)   B. ½ inch (1.25 cm)   C. ¼ inch (0.6 cm)

STUDENT'S NAME   DATE   GRADE

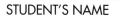
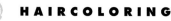

chart
degrees
groups formulation
level
saturation
stages

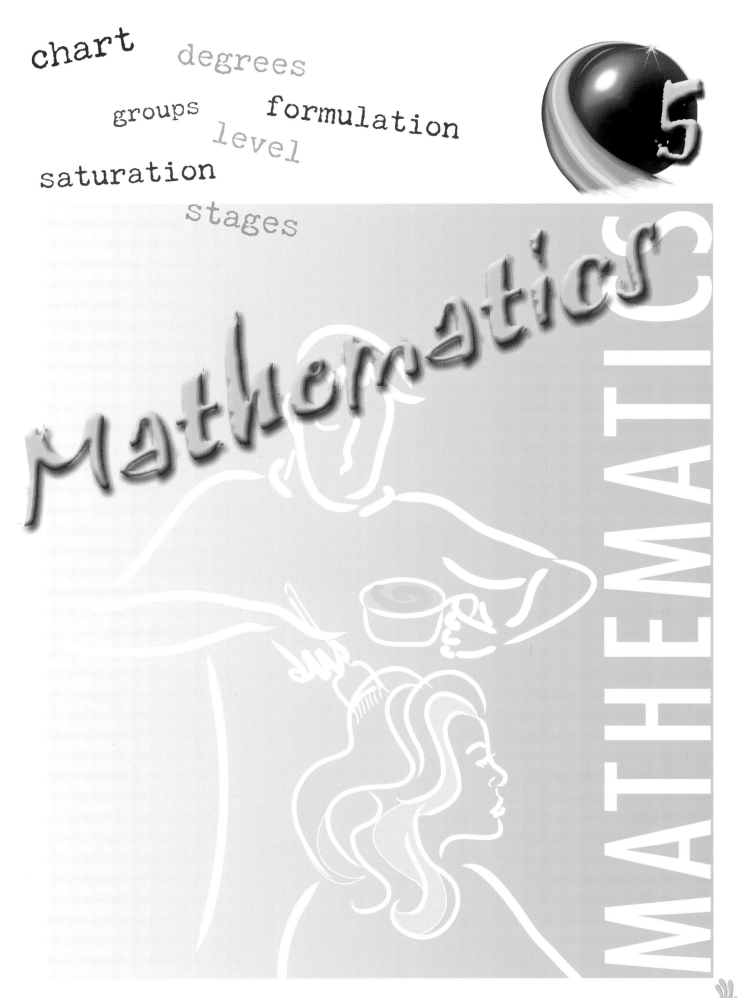

Mathematics

MATHEMATICS

Haircoloring Service ...

We apply mathematics in our everyday lives, whether we are at home baking a cake, attaching a shelf, at work itemizing materials or constructing a new house. As cosmetologists, we incorporate math when performing the client/guest consultation, deciding on the correct color shade for the client/guest, formulating the color mixture and even measuring the appropriate amount of color product for placement on the client/guest's hair.

Mathematics is the professional's connection to creating successful color results. Within the beauty industry, the basic math concepts of addition and subtraction – including counting, measuring, finding proportions, deciding the product quantity and percentages – are needed. This chapter will explore how the haircolorist applies those concepts during a client/guest consultation, when analyzing the client/guest's existing haircolor, selecting a color, formulating a color and applying the desired haircolor.

Sulfur

16

S

32.07

2.5

35.

The 9 Steps of Haircoloring...

The main areas of the haircoloring service are broken down into **nine major steps** for the professional to follow. Use these nine steps as your guide to make sure every part is successfully completed – this will result in a thorough color service. This chapter will offer a detailed explanation of each step, starting at the beginning of the color service to the final color result.

The 9 Steps of Haircoloring

1. Conduct a client/guest consultation

2. Perform a predisposition (patch) test

3. Determine the client/guest's natural/base haircolor level

4. Determine the client/guest's desired color shade/level

5. Determine the percent of white/gray hair

6. Determine color saturation/reflection

7. Create the color formula

8. Perform a strand test

9. Complete a client/guest record card (written or electronic) of the color service

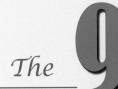

The U.S. Food, Drug and Cosmetic Act, states a predisposition (patch) test must be performed before each and every haircolor application. Check with your local regulatory agency if a predisposition (patch) test is administered 24 to 48 hours prior to the haircolor service.

Client / Guest Consultation ...

Step 1
Conduct a client/ guest consultation

The **consultation**, referred to as **"chair talk,"** is the first essential step of the haircoloring service. This is the cosmetologists' opportunity to ask questions and establish a relationship with the client/guest in order to get to know his or her hair-care needs and desired haircolor. To set up a consultation, **book an extra fifteen minutes prior** to the actual hair service. **Conduct the consultation in a properly lit area** of the salon; preferably in a room that emits natural light and if not, in an area where the walls are painted in neutral colors or plain white to help distinguish the most accurate natural haircolor.

The consultation is separated into two general areas:

Scalp and hair analysis is a **crucial area** and should never be overlooked…if the hair and scalp is not in a healthy state or a **disease is present, a haircolor service cannot be performed**… refer to a medical care professional.

NOTE: Refer to Chapter 4 (Biological Powers) for the detailed breakdown of the scalp and hair analysis.

● **First** –
Analyzing the hair and scalp

1.

● **Second** –
Agreeing on a desired haircolor and the placement of that color

2.

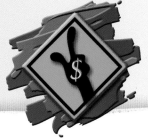

As the professional, help the client/guest to restore hair and/or scalp back to a healthy state by suggesting a series of reconditioning services. Also recommend hair-care products to use at home.

Client/Guest Consultation ...

When conducting a client/guest consultation, remember to apply the two components of people skills – **human relations and ethics. Human relations** is building a **relationship between you and the client/guest** by establishing good communication and listening skills. It is developing an understanding of the client/guest's needs and having a compassionate, caring attitude for each individual. **Ethics** are a person's **morals or beliefs** by which he or she lives and works. This is shown through a person's behavior toward others, such as being **courteous, helpful and respectful.** During and after the scalp and hair analysis, **ask a series of questions** to acquaint you with the client/guest's lifestyle and to build an understanding of his or hers hair-care needs. Below is a general set of questions to ask during the client/guest consultation. These are just a few questions: you are not limited to asking only these questions – ask as many questions necessary in order to move to the next part of the consultation.

Explore the hair-care needs and desires of the client/guest:

- What chemical hair services has the client/guest received in the last six months?

- If client/guest has artificial color, was it done professionally or is the color a store-bought haircolor?

- How much time does the client/guest spend or would like to spend on his or her hair each day? What styling aids are used on the hair?

- Does the client/guest participate in activities or sports such as swimming, running, bicycling, etc.?

- Does the client/guest receive other chemical services such as permanent waving or chemical relaxing?

- What does the client/guest like or dislike about his or her hair?

- A brief medical history. Is the client/guest on any daily medications? And if so, what are the medicines?

"As you continue your client/guest consultation, maintain good listening skills, as it is easy to get distracted by your own thoughts and ideas, which may make you forget to focus on what the client/guest is telling you!"

Compile these answers along with the scalp and hair analysis results on a client/guest record card. At this part of the client/guest consultation, the cosmetologist will know whether he or she can proceed with the remaining steps of the consultation.

Client/Guest Consultation ...

Before

After

1

Ask a separate set of questions to better acquaint you with the client/guest's **haircolor needs** and the procedure used to apply the color. Below is a general set of guidelines and questions to help narrow down the color choice and if it would be in the best interest for the client/guest.

- Present a portfolio with **before and after images** of models showcasing multiple color results and dimensional effects.

  - Carefully select **professional terms** to accentuate the positives and avoid any negative implications.

    For example, incorporate the following terms:

    - "lighten" instead of "bleach"
    - "remove" instead of "strip"
    - "new growth" or "regrowth," instead of "roots"
    - "refresh" instead of "touch-up"

  - Compare **client/guest's terminology with professional terminology. For example:**

    - When the client/guest asks for light blonde, does he or she really mean pastel blonde?

    - When the client/guest asks for auburn, does he or she really mean dark red?

  - Does the client/guest want a **temporary, semi-permanent, demi-permanent or permanent haircolor?** Explain maintenance for all categories of colors.

Client / Guest Consultation ...

- Is he or she interested in an **over-all color application** or **coloring selected strands of hair** (highlight or lowlight)?

- Is the client/guest wanting the end color result to be conservative or would he or she rather have a **dramatic finish?**

- Briefly **paraphrase your understanding** of the client/guest's requests and desired end color results.

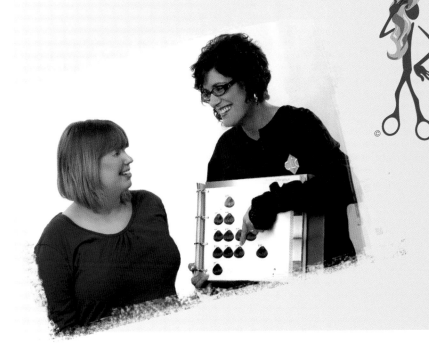

"Remember your own appearance as a stylist is an advertisement for your haircoloring services. Creating great effects with your own haircolor will go a long way toward building your credibility and marketing haircolor services!"

Client/Guest Consultation ...

At this part of the consultation, deliver your **suggestions** on what you feel would be more **appropriate for the client/guest.** Explain the facts on how your recommendations will benefit his or her lifestyle, enhance appearance, and help with the client/guest's maintenance and hair-care needs.

Suggest and explain your recommendations to the client/guest.

● Suggest more than one option for the client/guest's haircolor request. Show images of people that wear the same color to support your recommendation.

● Describe how the recommended haircolor can be used to accentuate the positive features and/or diminish the less positive features. It can also be used to accentuate part of a hairstyle or haircut.

Client/Guest Consultation ...

● Explain the details of the color procedure (be honest), cost of color service and cost of visits to maintain the haircolor. Cost and maintenance may be deciding factors if the client/guest will accept your recommendation.

RELEASE STATEMENT

I, the undersigned, (client/guest's name) _____ live at _____ and am about to
(street, city, state and zip code) _____ at the (salon or school name) _____
receive (chemical service name) _____ .

I, (client/guest's name) _____ was advised of the possible risks to
my hair and scalp during the chemical service performed on (date) _____ and the
service fees by either students, graduate students, and/or educators, or professionals of the
school or salon establishment.

I, (client/guest's name) _____ hereby release the salon, school
or professional establishment and professionals, students, and/or educators therein from any and
all claims that may occur during and in any way connected with the delivery of the particular
chemical service.

The owner of professional establishment is not responsible for personal property.

_____
_____
*Signed _____
Date _____
Manager or Owner _____

*If client /guest being serviced is under 18 years of age, he or she
will need a parent or guardian to sign release form.

● Some salons require a release statement before providing any chemical services. This is required for some salon malpractice insurance policies. Be sure to get a signed release if client/guest is insisting on receiving the color service despite your recommendations not to get the service (refer to page 151).

● Politely decline a haircolor request from your client/guest if you feel the service will damage the hair. Be prepared to thoroughly explain your reasons as to why you will not perform the service.

CLIENT/GUEST RECORD CARD

Name _____

Address _____ Date _____

Home Phone _____ Work _____ Mobile _____

Email Address _____

Birthdate (month/day)_____ Occupation _____

First Visit Date _____

Check all that apply:

Medications __ Allergies __

Personal Hair-Care Products: Shampoo __ Conditioner __ Hairspray __ Gel __Other __

Professional Haircoloring: Temporary __ Semi-Permanent __ Demi-Permanent __

Permanent __ Lightener __ Home Haircolor __

I receive the following chemical services: Color __ Perm __ Lightening __ Relaxer__

Cosmetologist _____ License # _____

Hair Condition: Normal __ Dry __ Breakage __   Scalp Condition: Normal __ Dry __ Oily __

Texture: Fine __ Medium __ Coarse __

Density: Thick __ Medium __ Thin __   Type of Hair: Straight __ Wavy __ Curly __

Porosity: Resistant __ Normal __ Severe __ Irregular __

Elasticity: Average __ Low __

Length: Short __ Medium __ Long __

Patch Test Administered: Date/Initials Examined: Date/Initials

Results: Positive __ Negative __

What attracted you to our salon? Friend __ Location __ Advertisement __

REMARKS _____

B A C K

Client/Guest Haircolor Level: Natural ___ Desired ___ Percentage of Gray_____
Haircolor Formulation:_____
Timing:_____
First Time Color Results: _____
Retouch Color Formulation: _____
Retouch Results:_____
Service Date with Cost:_____

DATE	SERVICE/TREATMENT-Formula/Product/Procedure	REMARKS/CHANGES

CLIENT/GUEST RECORD CARD

Name _____ Date _____ Cosmetologist _____ License # _____
Address _____ Hair Condition: Normal __Dry __ Breakage __   Scalp Condition: Normal __ Dry __ Oily __
Home Phone _____ Work _____ Mobile _____ Texture: Fine __ Medium __ Coarse __ Type of Hair: Straight __ Wavy __ Curly __
Email Address _____ Density: Thick __ Medium __ Thin __
Birthdate (month/day)_____ Occupation _____ Porosity: Resistant __ Normal __ Severe __ Irregular __
First Visit Date _____ Elasticity: Average __ Low __   Length: Short __ Medium __ Long __
Patch Test Administered: Date/Initials Examined: Date/Initials
Check all that apply: Results: Positive __ Negative __
Medications __ Allergies __ What attracted you to our salon? Friend __ Location __ Advertisement __
Personal Hair-Care Products: Shampoo __ Conditioner __ Hairspray __ Gel __Other __ REMARKS _____
Professional Haircoloring: Temporary __ Semi-Permanent __ Demi-Permanent __
Permanent __ Lightener __ Home Haircolor __
I receive the following chemical services: Color __ Perm __ Lightening __ Relaxer__

Keeping accurate client/guest records of services rendered is only half of the job ... recording the cost of services is the other half!

Release Statement ...

W henever there is possible risk of impairing a client/guest's hair during a chemical service the client/guest is recommended **not** to receive the service, but he or she insists on getting the service regardless of the consequences, *a release statement is issued for the client/guest to read and sign. A **release statement** is a form **affirming that the client/guest** was advised of the potential risks that could result during the requested chemical service.*

Keep in mind, a release statement is **not a required legal form and would not clear** the school/student/professional of the responsibility to deliver a successful hair service. For the best interest of the school or salon and all involved, if the student or the professional has any doubt about performing the requested service to his or her best ability, then **please decline the service and suggest other hair-care service alternatives.**

RELEASE STATEMENT

I, the undersigned, (client/guest's name) _____ live at _____ and am about to
(street, city, state and zip code) _____ at the (salon or school name) _____.
receive (chemical service name) _____

I, (client/guest's name) _____ was advised of the possible risks to
my hair and/or scalp during the chemical service performed on (date) _____ and the
service fees by either students, graduate students, and/or educators, or professionals of the
school or salon establishment.

I, (client/guest's name) _____ hereby release the salon, school
or professional establishment and professionals, students, and/or educators therein from any and
all claims that may occur during and in any way connected with the delivery of the particular
chemical service.

The owner of this professional establishment is not responsible for personal property.

*Signed _____
Date _____
Manager or Owner _____

*If client being serviced is under 18 years of age, he or she
will need a parent or guardian to sign release form.

Disclaimer: *The release form shown is an example and not to be duplicated for your own personal salon or school use.*

Predisposition Testing ...

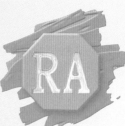

Step Two
Perform a predisposition (patch) test

Allergy is a **hypersensitivity response** to a normally harmless substance to which the body reacts. It is an antigen-antibody disorder, reaction or extreme sensitivity to chemicals, drugs, foods, animals and other substances. It is impossible to predict whether an individual will experience an allergic reaction to haircolor, therefore a **predisposition or patch test is an important step prior to any haircoloring service.**

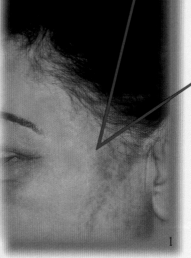

1

According to the **U.S. Food, Drug and Cosmetic Act, a predisposition (patch) test must be performed before each and every haircolor application.**

Predisposition or patch test is applying a small amount of the haircolor mixture on the skin to check for skin sensitivity of product/chemical. Any haircolor containing **aniline derivative tint** requires a patch test be given **24 to 48 hours prior to haircolor service**. Each haircolor product label displays a warning, advertising to perform patch test prior to haircolor service. Always check with the haircolor manufacturer on the requisites when patch testing.

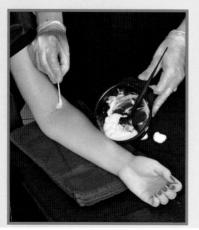

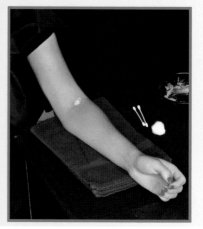

Predisposition Testing...

The patch test can be administered on two areas of the body, either **behind the ear extending into the hairline, or innerfold of elbow.** Always record the date of the predisposition test and results on the client/guest record card for future reference. Refer to Chapter 6 for actual patch test procedure.

Two Patch Test Reactions:

1 **-** **Negative** – there is **NO sensitivity** to the haircolor product

2 **+** **Positive** – **there is a sensitivity** to the haircolor product; recognized by **rash, hives, swelling and inflammation.** If one or more of these symptoms occur, seek a medical care professional. Severe reactions are trouble breathing, swallowing and thickness of tongue or blistering of skin.

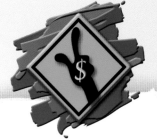

The salon may save money on its insurance policy if the cosmetologist takes the legal and precautionary measures by giving a patch test prior to all haircoloring services.

CAUTION: **DO NOT** apply aniline derivative (coal tar dyes) tint to eyelashes and eyebrows – this may cause blindness. Use a color product that is especially designed for tinting the eyebrows and lashes, if permitted by your local regulatory agency.

Natural Haircolor Level ...

3

Step Three

Determine the client/guest's natural or base haircolor level

*An individual's natural or base haircolor is derived from the **melanocyte cells located in the cortex layer** of the hair. Each client/guest has a unique arrangement of melanin granules, which develop the dimensions of color. The hue (tone), level and intensity of a color determine an individual's natural haircolor. It is important to know that not every client/guest will respond to a specific haircolor the same way, therefore analyzing the client/guest's natural level of color is the first step in deciding the color to be used.*

Natural haircolor basically ranges in shades from **black, brown, red and blonde.** The color is broken down into levels and each level is given a number from 1 to 10.

Level or value is determining the **degree of lightness or darkness of a color** depending on how much light is reflected or absorbed. **Low numbers are the dark colors** (levels 1 to 3), **middle numbers are the medium colors** (levels 4 to 7) and **high numbers are the light shades** (levels 8 to 10).

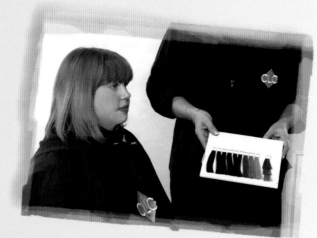

For example:

| Number 1 Black | Number 5 Medium Brown | Number 7 Medium Blonde | Number 10 Lightest Blonde |

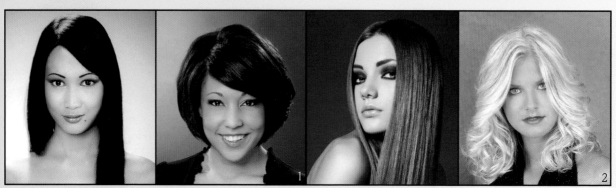

Disclaimer: *It is important to note that the level systems will vary greatly depending on the haircolor manufacturer of choice. Some level system numbering will range from 1 to 12 or go as high as 1 to 16, but the universal range is 1 to 10. Carefully read the manufacturer's instructions before formulating a haircolor mixture.*

Natural Haircolor Level...

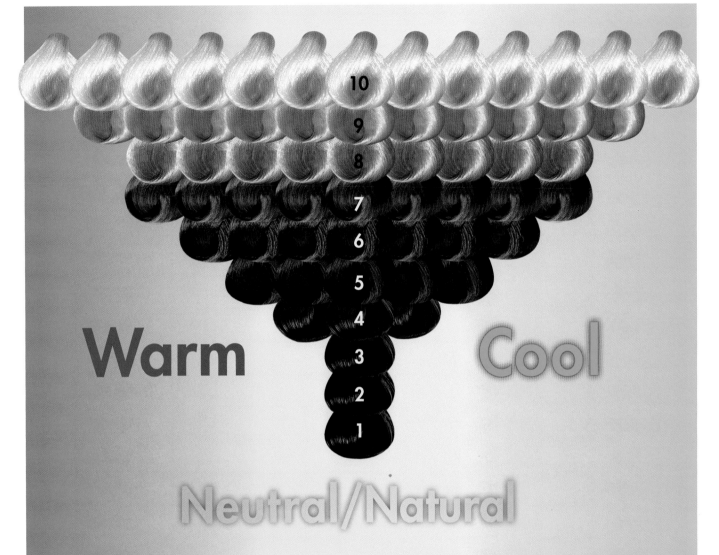

Warm   Cool

10
9
8
7
6
5
4
3
2
1

Neutral/Natural

Another area that is distinguishable on the level system is the tone or temperature of a color. Color tones generally start at a level 4 and are separated into warm, cool and neutral.

Colors classified as warm tones are **red, yellow, orange or golden,** which are typically referred to as copper, auburn, bronze, strawberry or amber colors to a client/guest.

Colors classified as cool tones are **blue, green and violet,** known as ash, drab or smoky colors.

Colors considered neutral are the **natural colors.**

Haircolor Families ...

*M*ost professional haircolor manufacturers *will display their haircolors on hair swatches placed in a* **chart or binder.** *Every manufacturer will design and identify its haircolors differently ... the level numbering and color identification will vary. It is very important to study the salon's haircolor system for directions in how to use and apply the haircolor product. Most manufacturers will* **offer educational seminars** *or have a representative that provides classes periodically throughout the year. This is a great way for the new employee to learn about the color system and to keep the existing employees abreast on new information. As stated before, the information in this book is a basic overview, and is to be used as a foundation to learning the principles and art of haircoloring.*

On a haircolor swatch chart, the color hues and intensities are separated into groups referred to as **series or families,** which are then identified by a "letter." The shade divisions help the haircolorist when performing color services in the salon.

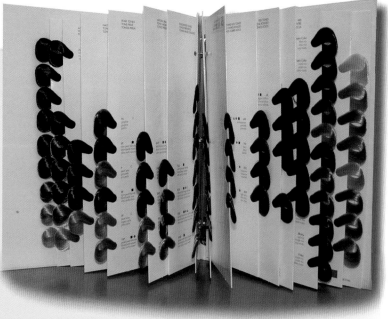

Haircolor Families or Series

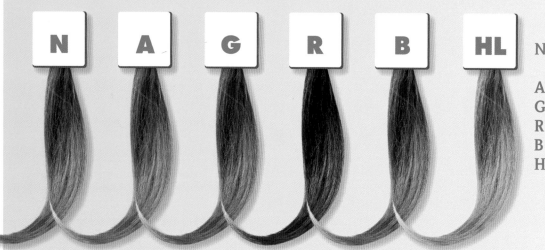

N – Neutral or
Natural Series
A – Ash Series
G – Gold Series
R – Red Series
B – Beige Series
HL – High-Lift
Blonde Series

Haircolor Families ...

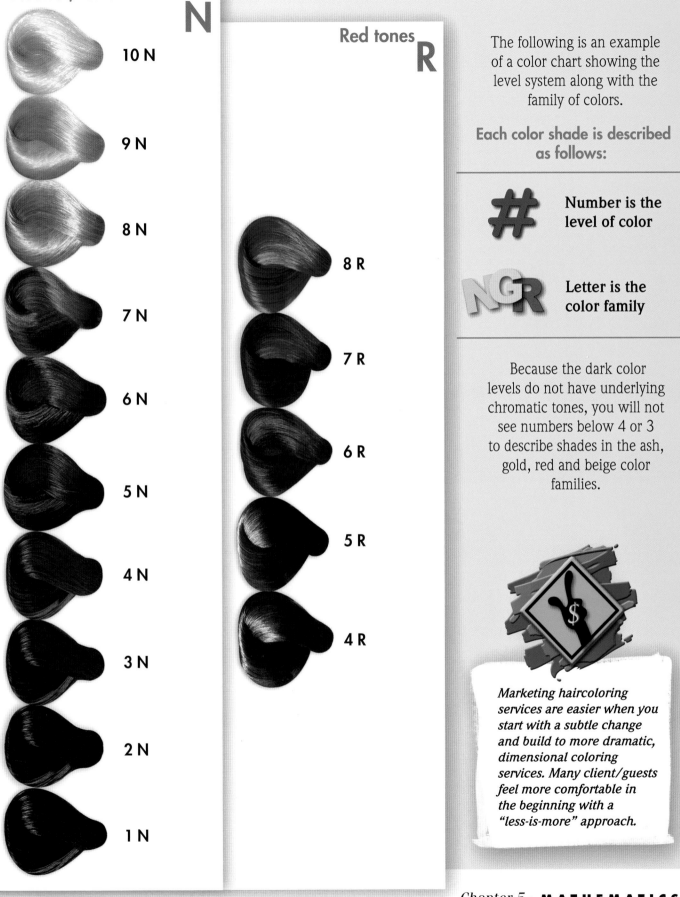

Neutral/Natural tones
N

10 N
9 N
8 N
7 N
6 N
5 N
4 N
3 N
2 N
1 N

Red tones
R

8 R
7 R
6 R
5 R
4 R

The following is an example of a color chart showing the level system along with the family of colors.

Each color shade is described as follows:

Number is the level of color

N G R   Letter is the color family

Because the dark color levels do not have underlying chromatic tones, you will not see numbers below 4 or 3 to describe shades in the ash, gold, red and beige color families.

Marketing haircoloring services are easier when you start with a subtle change and build to more dramatic, dimensional coloring services. Many client/guests feel more comfortable in the beginning with a "less-is-more" approach.

Family Heritage ...

Because today's population is a **melting pot of diverse heritages,** each individual's hair will respond slightly different to haircolor. For optimal results, it is important to determine your client/guest's original ethnic heritage prior to developing the color formulation you will use. There are seven basic "families" of hair, based upon broad multi-cultural descriptions. The chart on the next page will explain each family heritage with the typical haircolor, skin tone, eye color, and ancestry and color formulation ranges.

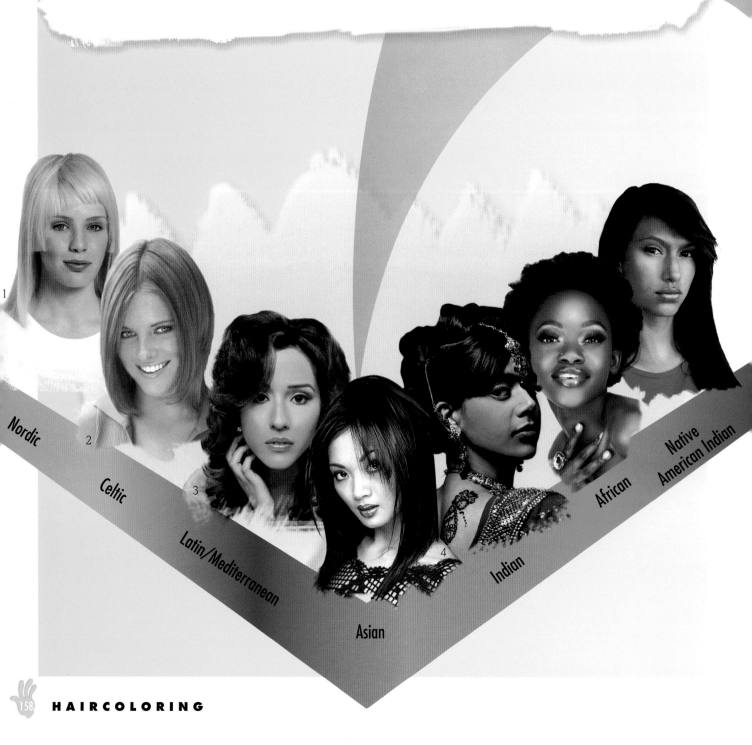

1

Nordic

2

Celtic

3

Latin/Mediterranean

Asian

4

Indian

African

Native American Indian

Family Heritage ...

Families of Hair	Range of Natural Color Level	Skin Tone	Eye Color	Family Background	Range of Formulation
Nordic	6 to 10	Pale without pink tones	Light blue or gray	**Scandinavian, Norwegian, German, Slavic or Danish.** Haircolor has little to no natural warmth. Any desired color is easy to achieve. Warm to gold undertones.	Four levels of lift are possible using standard permanent color. Cool ashen tones and soft golden shades of beiges are more flattering. Level 5 or darker is not as flattering.
Celtic	4 to 7	Light with gold or pink undertones and often with freckles	Deep or bright blue, green, hazel or golden brown	**Northern European — Irish, Scottish, Dutch and Welsh.** Hair has gold undertones. Irish has red undertones.	Three levels of lift are possible using standard permanent color. More lift will show gold or red undertones. Golden blondes, honey beiges, red, red-copper are pleasing.
Latin/ Mediterranean	3 to 6	Olive with yellow undertones	Hazel, green or brown	**Southern European — Italian, Greek, French, Spanish, South American Borderline — Iranian, Israeli, Egyptian, Turkish.** A large degree of iron is present in this hair type, which produces red tones when lightening hair.	Only two levels of lift are possible using standard permanent color. Avoid ash colors and encourage vibrant reds, red-violets, warm and gold colors.
Asian	1 to 4	Pale with strong yellow tones	Dark brown	**Japanese, Chinese, Korean, Vietnamese, Thai, Cambodian, Mongolian and Malaysian —** High density of melanin and very tight, compact cuticle scales.	Dark red and golds, chestnuts and coffee shades are flattering. Lightening this type of hair is challenging.
Indian	1 to 3	Brown	Dark brown	**Indian (country of India) —** Soft, fine hair, generally will gray earlier in life. Hair has warm undertones.	Dark to medium brown with red to gold highlights. Avoid lightening this hair.
African Natural color level, skin and eye color will vary greatly	1 to 4	Varying levels of brown/black	Dark brown	**African, Egyptian and Moroccan —** Hair has a natural curl and is often very porous through previous chemical services. Hair has red undertones.	General rule of thumb — levels 6 and lower will deposit color and levels 7 and up will lift on natural levels. Strand testing is recommended.
Native American	1 to 3	Red	Dark brown	**North and South American —** Strong hair and the darkest of all families of hair. Hair has red undertones.	Dark shades of black, brown and dark reds.

Eye Pigmentation

As the chart indicates on the previous page, eye color is another source for determining an individual's heritage (background) and natural haircolor. As a general rule of thumb, decide under which pigmentation group the eye color falls by following the information below.

The two basic groups of eye pigmentation are iron or sulfur.

IRON PIGMENTS

People with dark color eyes have iron pigmentation. The original ancestry was dominant in **eumelanin, which produces black pigments.** This group includes Latino, Mediterranean, Asian, African, Indian, Native American Indian, Eskimo and Middle Eastern people. When lifting the natural haircolor to lighter shades, a red undertone will appear in the hair.

People with sulfur pigmentation have light eyes.
The original ancestry was either dominant in eumelanin or dominant in pheomelanin, thereby producing red and yellow pigments. Or they had a combination of eumelanin and pheomelanin (mixed melanin) producing red, yellow, brown and black pigments. This group has yellow undertones and when going lighter than the natural haircolor, the yellow color will come through.

Sometimes due to the many diverse cultures and ancestry, evaluating a person's eye color may not produce the most accurate reading when deciding on the natural haircolor. Further questioning and evaluating is necessary in order to make the closest accurate assessment.

Sulfer Pigments

"Always strand test when unsure of the natural underlying pigment."

When deciding the client/guest's natural or base level color, always view his or her hair in the **best possible light source** such as natural light. If natural light is not available (rain or cloudy day), halogen or LED lighting is the next best choice. The haircolorist's objective is to **determine the client/guest's level of darkness to lightness** – concentration of pigment in the hair.

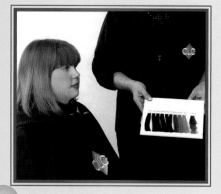

1 Use the color chart; refer to the natural/neutral color series hair swatches.

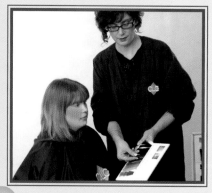

2 Select a hair swatch that closely resembles the client/guest's natural level.

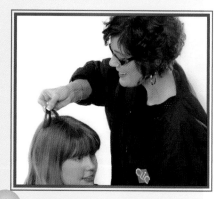

3 Position and spread hair swatch into the scalp area, resting on the hair.

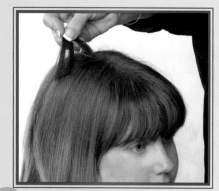

4 Hair swatch should blend into the natural haircolor – **Reminder:** you are deciding on concentration of pigment (level), not family of color.

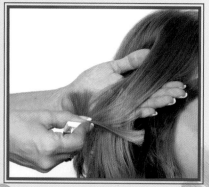

5 Choose a different color series and hair swatch level to decide the color level on the mid-strand.

NOTE: If the color appears to fall between two levels, choose the darkest level.

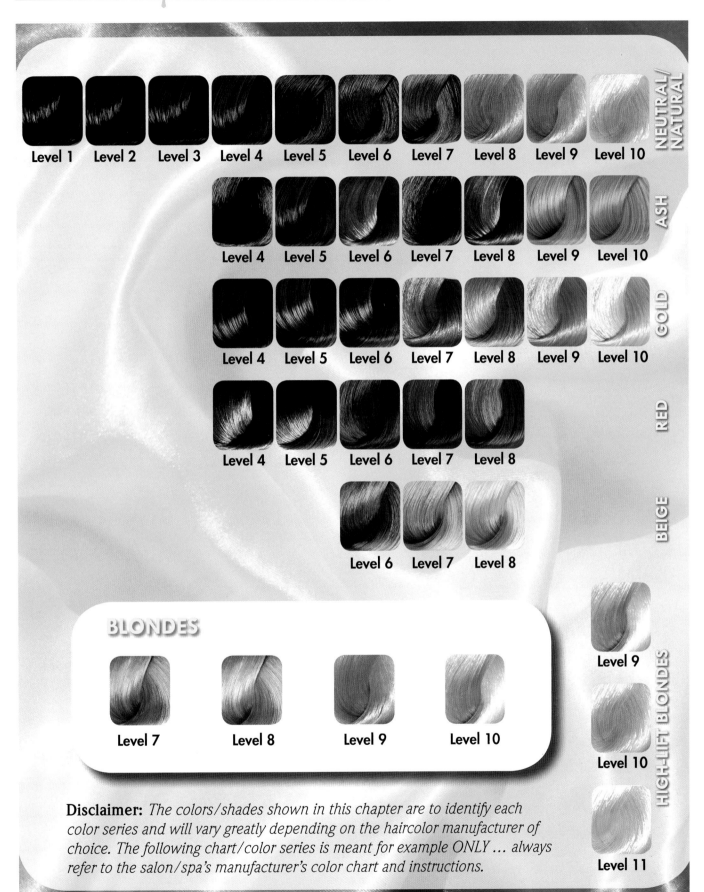

NEUTRAL/NATURAL

Level 1   Level 2   Level 3   Level 4   Level 5   Level 6   Level 7   Level 8   Level 9   Level 10

ASH

Level 4   Level 5   Level 6   Level 7   Level 8   Level 9   Level 10

GOLD

Level 4   Level 5   Level 6   Level 7   Level 8   Level 9   Level 10

RED

Level 4   Level 5   Level 6   Level 7   Level 8

BEIGE

Level 6   Level 7   Level 8

BLONDES

Level 7   Level 8   Level 9   Level 10

HIGH-LIFT BLONDES

Level 9

Level 10

Level 11

Disclaimer: *The colors/shades shown in this chapter are to identify each color series and will vary greatly depending on the haircolor manufacturer of choice. The following chart/color series is meant for example ONLY ... always refer to the salon/spa's manufacturer's color chart and instructions.*

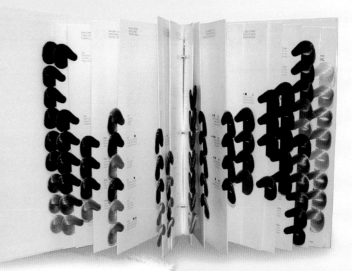

Step Four
Determine the client/guest's desired color shade/level

The client/guest will use a haircolor chart to select the desired level and color of his or her liking. Since every manufacturer has its own haircolor chart, the professional is required to study and learn each color family along with its recommended use. Most color manufacturers will offer classes, which are conducted by a product representative, who educates the professionals on how to use a particular manufacturer's haircolor system.

The following is a breakdown of each color series from a standard haircolor chart *(this is only an example)*:

NATURAL/NEUTRAL

is a blend of all **three primary colors, but in unequal proportions,** resulting in more natural shades. This series is available in **10 levels – level 1 (blue black) to level 10 (lightest blonde).** The neutral family is used when determining the natural level of hair. If the hair falls between two levels, choose the darkest one. To color gray hair, the neutral series may be used alone or added to another color family to provide the best coverage. Neutral shades will soften natural highlights or any remaining tones left in the hair.

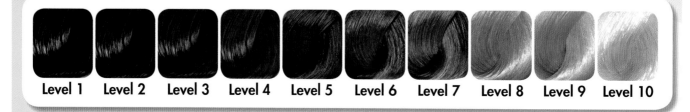

Level 1   Level 2   Level 3   Level 4   Level 5   Level 6   Level 7   Level 8   Level 9   Level 10

Identify Desired Color Level ...

◤ ASH

is **unequal mixtures of blue and violet base shades** with no primary yellow, which are arranged in **levels of 4 to 10.** The ash family is used to minimize brassy or unwanted orange and red tones. Ash colors are **not recommended** for pure white hair or when covering gray hair. For gray or "salt and pepper" hair, the ash would tone down the gray color as the white hair would change to silver. The ash colors appear drab and usually develop to a dark level more so than any other family of color.

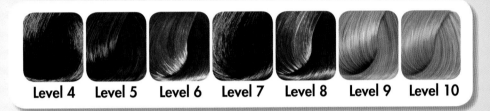

◤ GOLD

colors consist of **red and yellow** with yellow being the predominant tone. This family of color is available in **levels 4 to 10,** providing **soft golden shades.** The gold series is highly recommended for gray coverage because yellow and red are the two primary colors missing from gray hair. The gold colors may successfully be mixed with red, neutral, beige or red-violet color families.

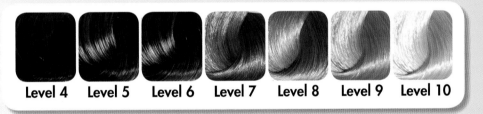

◤ RED

series has varying red colors with either a **base of yellow (warm) or a base of violet (cool).** The red series ranges from **levels 4 to 8** and generally falls under the red-violet or red-orange category. It is recommended not to use the red series by itself when covering gray, but it can be added to the color formulation to produce warm tonal values.

- **Red flame** has a base of red and yellow with strong red tones
- **Red copper** is a mixture of red and yellow in unequal proportions
- **Red-violet** consists of a mixture of red and blue
- **Red-orange** contains a red and yellow base with predominant orange tones

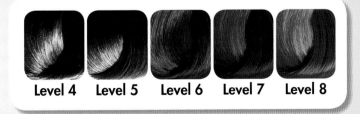

BEIGE

is a **blend of red, yellow and blue** with less intensity than the natural/neutral family. The beige family is available in **levels 6 to 8.** This color series provides excellent coverage for gray hair while adding the tones that are generally missing in the gray color. It is also excellent when mixed with the red and gold families of color.

- **Nordic beige** is a base of red, yellow and blue with a high concentration of blue
- **Honey beige** consists of unequal proportions of red, yellow (predominant tone) and blue with a trace of violet

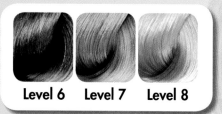

Level 6   Level 7   Level 8

BLONDE

consists of **unequal proportions of red, yellow and blue with a high concentration of yellow.** The blonde series ranges from **level 7 to 10 or higher** depending on manufacturer. Any level darker than a 7 level will need to be decolorized before applying a toner color.

- **Platinum blonde** has a blue and violet base
- **Pink blonde** has a hint of red, blue, violet and some yellow
- **Silver blonde** has a base of red, yellow, blue (blue is predominant) and some violet

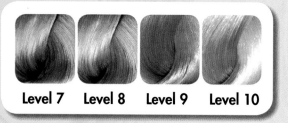

Level 7   Level 8   Level 9   Level 10

HIGH-LIFT BLONDES include the families of ash, beige, gold and natural. High-lift blondes are designed to increase lightness in naturally colored hair having more control in a one-step process. In order to be able to **lift four or more levels,** high-lift colors are mixed with either a 30 or 40 volume developer, but always check with the color manufacturer.

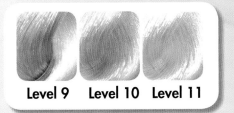

Level 9   Level 10   Level 11

"High-lift blondes work best when only lightening up to three levels; otherwise a double process would be considered ... pre-lightening and toning the hair."

5

Step Five
Determine the amount of white/gray hair

*S*ince the amount of melanin *in each individual hair is unpredictable throughout our lifetime, it is an important step to determine if the client/guest has any gray or white hair.* **Gray hair** *is the result of a* **gradual or slowing down of melanin** *production in the cortex layer of the hair. Generally, most client/guests will have a percentage of gray hair; meaning a combination of pigmented (gray) hair and non-pigmented (white) hair, referred to as "salt and pepper" hair. Using the chart below as your guide, perform an overview of the entire client/guest's head to decide the percentage of gray.*

Gray Hair Percentage

Level System	25 Percent – more gray hair, less white hair	50 Percent – an equal mixture of gray and white hair	75 Percent – less gray hair, more white hair
LIGHT	25%	50%	75%
MEDIUM	25%	50%	75%
DARK	25%	50%	75%

NOTE: Gray hair still contains the three primary colors, but in **unequal amounts.** Blue is the predominant color, which eventually fades, resulting in light shades of gray. In some rare occurrences, all of the client/guest's hair may be a solid gray, with no combination of white and gray hair.

When hair has a **total absence of pigment** – no eumelanin or pheomelanin, it is referred to as **white hair.**

Location of gray hair is another area of consideration when determining the gray's percentage. Generally gray hair will begin at the **sideburns, front hairline or top and crown of head.** It is suggested to apply the color mixture in these areas first to ensure proper color absorption.

Gray Hair Coverage ...

Due to the varying concentrations of pigment in gray hair, **certain factors** must be considered when formulating for gray coverage. Keep in mind the haircolorist is dealing with **some hair strands containing little to no pigment, while there are other hair strands that contain pigment.** Another area to take into account is gray hair may react differently when a **light shade of color** is desired. High color levels (level 8 and up) might not completely cover the gray hair due to a **low pigment** concentration in the color itself, whereas medium to dark levels of color will cover gray easier because there is a higher concentration of pigment.

Factors to consider when using semi-permanent or demi-permanent haircolor

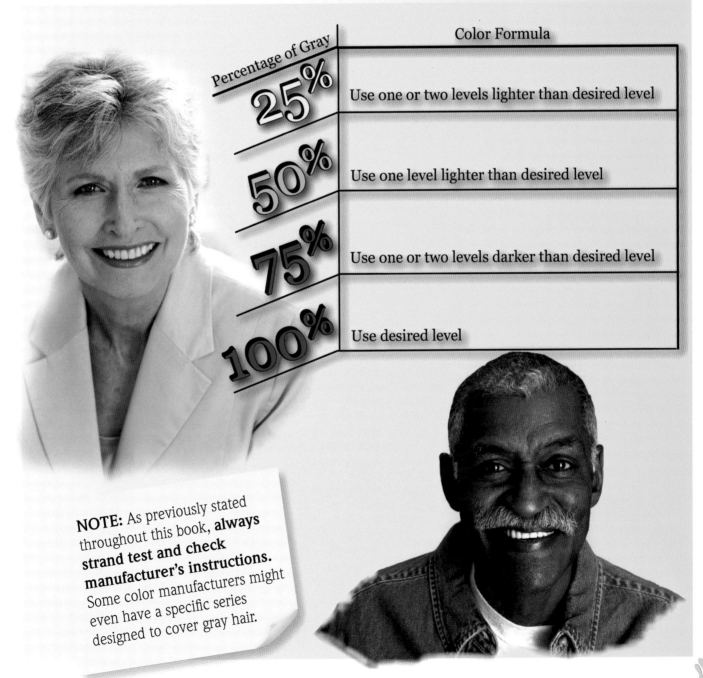

Percentage of Gray	Color Formula
25%	Use one or two levels lighter than desired level
50%	Use one level lighter than desired level
75%	Use one or two levels darker than desired level
100%	Use desired level

NOTE: As previously stated throughout this book, **always strand test and check manufacturer's instructions.** Some color manufacturers might even have a specific series designed to cover gray hair.

Gray Hair Coverage ...

Factors to consider when using permanent haircolor:

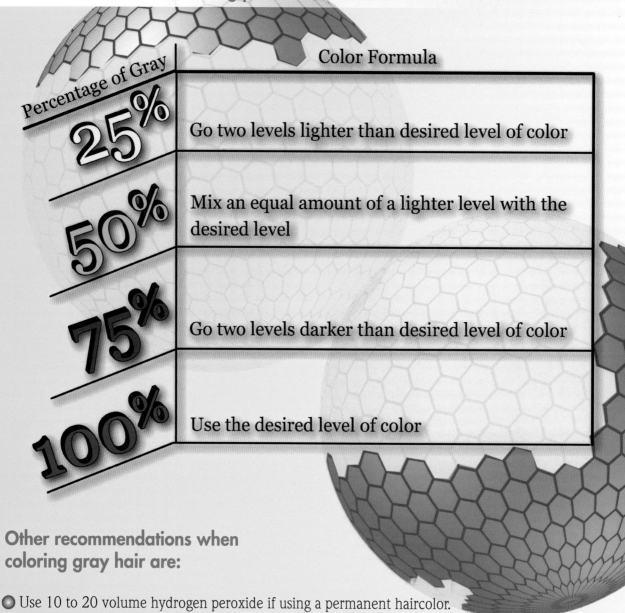

Percentage of Gray	Color Formula
25%	Go two levels lighter than desired level of color
50%	Mix an equal amount of a lighter level with the desired level
75%	Go two levels darker than desired level of color
100%	Use the desired level of color

Other recommendations when coloring gray hair are:

- Use 10 to 20 volume hydrogen peroxide if using a permanent haircolor.

- Include in color formula a warm or natural/neutral series to assist in covering gray (an ash series will not successfully cover gray hair).

- Process color the full development time following manufacturer's instructions.

- To create a very light blonde, lift to a level 7 followed by a highlight application.

Reminder: The **ash series** can make gray hair appear cool or drab and **may not cover the gray hair completely,** especially if it is a high percentage of gray. Always check with the color manufacturer for information on how its ash-based colors perform, since each color line is manufactured differently.

Gray hair is sometimes **resistant to color absorption** because of the compact cuticle scales and the extra layers of cuticle scales. **Resistant** is when a chemical, in this case haircolor, does not penetrate into the cuticle and cortex layers of the hair within a relative amount of time to develop the color. **Porosity** is the absorption of liquid into the hair, which is determined by the condition of the cuticle. Perform a strand test to decide if the client/guest's gray hair is resistant to the absorption of haircolor.

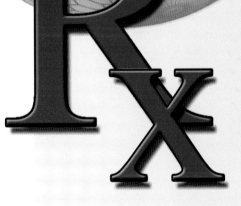

Pre-softening is when a product is placed on the resistant areas to "initiate" the process of opening the cuticle scales, which allows equal absorption. This can be performed in different ways – some color lines have their own **pre-softening product,** which is applied, processed and removed. While other manufacturers have you mix the **desired color with distilled water** and apply to only the resistant area(s) … process, gently blot excess color from hair and then re-apply a fresh mixture of color over entire head, including the resistant hair. Some resistant areas are the sideburns, temples and crown, which may appear as spots or streaks.

Yellowing hair is caused by staining, which sometimes occurs on gray or white hair if a person **smokes,** has excessive **sun exposure,** or takes certain **medications** and/or has a buildup of **styling aids.** Use haircolor remover to get rid of any yellow stains before applying the haircolor formula.

Disclaimer: *The information we provide is a general synopsis for coloring gray hair along with some industry suggestions on its coverage. Depending on the salon's haircolor product of choice, we strongly recommend you read the manufacturer's instructions for its gray hair formulation and always perform a strand test.*

Color Saturation / Reflection ...

6

Step Six
Determine color saturation/ reflection

Color saturation works in conjunction with color intensity. It is a combination of pigment concentration and light reflection that results in a multitude of colors. Oxidative haircolor **is mixed with an oxidizing agent** such as hydrogen peroxide (acidic), which allows it the ability to either darken or lighten the hair. Permanent oxidative colors will also **contain alkalizing agents** such as ammonia to assist in color saturation and/or reflection.

Each color varies in its color saturation/reflection due to the amount of alkalizing agents in each bottle/tube of color. The **greater amount** of alkalizing agents in the color, **more color reflection** is achieved with **less color saturation** ... hence, **high levels of color** are produced. The **less amount** of alkalizing agents in the color, the **less color reflection** is achieved with **more color saturation** ... therefore; **low levels of color** are produced.

There is an inverse relationship between the lifting and depositing. In other words, **low levels of color have a low ratio** of alkalizing agents, and **high levels of color have a high ratio** of alkalizing agents.

2.5%

6% **4%**

Some color manufacturers will modify the lifting and depositing effects of haircolor by using different volumes of hydrogen peroxide. **High percentages of** H_2O will create **light levels,** whereas **low volumes of hydrogen peroxide** provide **dark levels** of color.

Alkalizing Agent Concentrations:

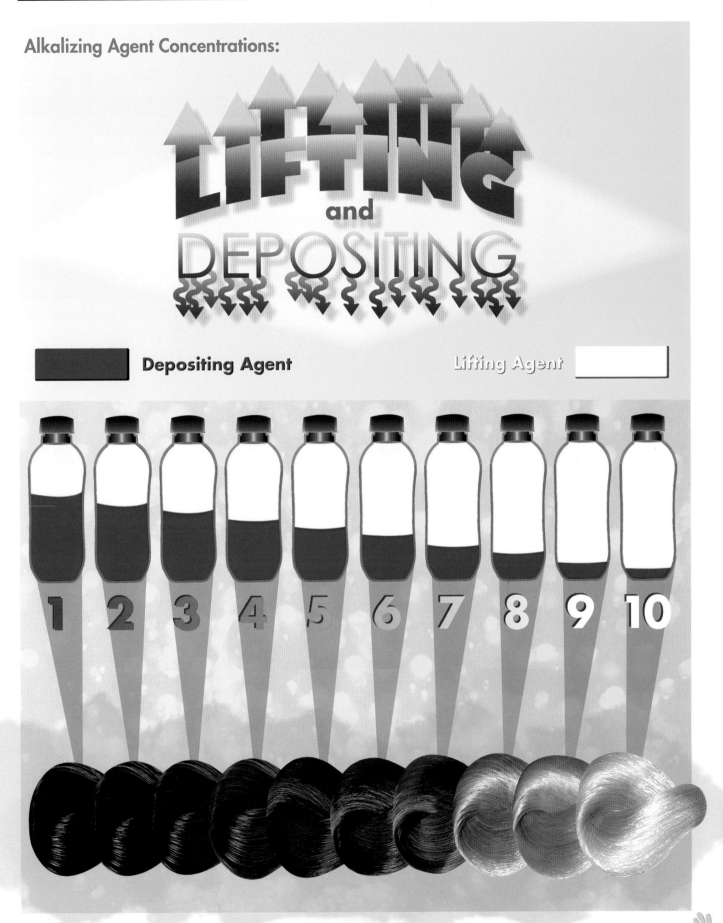

LIFTING and **DEPOSITING**

Depositing Agent

Lifting Agent

Haircolor Formulating ...

Step Seven
Create the color formula

*Color formulating is a standard four-part approach when determining the actual color formula/mixture used on the client/guest's hair. Keep in mind each area is **a basic guideline** to follow when introducing color formulating. However, **one and two are a necessary part when formulating** with any haircolor manufacturer, but as is stressed numerous times, always read color manufacturer's instructions first before proceeding with haircoloring service.*

Color Formulating:

1. Determine client/guest's natural or base level from the color manufacturer's color chart using the natural series.

2. Choose the client/guest's desired color, which includes the color's level, family and tonality of color.

3. If present, determine percentage of gray – use salt (white hair) and pepper (pigmented hair) as your guide. **Example:** If you see more pepper than salt, client/guest is **under 50 percent** gray. If there is an **equal amount** of salt and pepper, client/guest is 50 percent gray. If client/guest is **more** salt than pepper, client/guest is **above 50 percent** gray and when client/guest has **no** pepper, but all salt, he or she is 100 percent white.

   NOTE: Always read manufacturer's instructions of haircolor product used in the salon before formulating and applying any type of haircolor.

4. **Decide the volume/percentages of hydrogen peroxide used to create the color formula.** Some color manufacturers use developer volumes/percentages to produce the level of lift desired ... refer to the following page for more information on this type of formulating.

Haircolor Formulating...

When creating the desired haircolor by using various developer volumes/ percentages, use the chart below as your guide.

Reminder: This chart is an example; please follow manufacturer's instructions of the haircolor product being used in the salon for formulating and mixing.

10   20   30   40

Ten Volumes/3% H_2O_2	Twenty Volumes/6% H_2O_2	Thirty Volumes/9% H_2O_2	Forty Volumes/12% H_2O_2
For going darker than natural/base level	For depositing at base level	For going two levels lighter than natural/base level	Going three levels lighter than base level
Use for toning pre-lightened hair	Going one level lighter than natural/base level	Going three levels lighter using an intensifier (check manufacturer's directions)	Going four levels lighter using an intensifier (check manufacturer's directions)
	For optimum gray coverage		

In haircoloring, always **use caution when trying to reach three to four levels of lightness with oxidative haircolor.** Some color levels range from 1 to 12 or higher – check with color manufacturer to see if this is achievable without using a lightener. If lightener (bleach) is needed to achieve the level of lightness desired, there are two options available to the client/guest; double process (complete lightener application followed by toner) or off-the-scalp services (foiling or cap highlighting).

"Do not forget to double-check liquid H_2O_2 volume strength by using a hydrometer."

Haircolor Formulating ...

Undertone is the underlying or base color seen within the predominant color. It can be a result of the natural inborn pigments, or artificially created to produce a two-level effect.

If wanting to counterbalance the natural inborn or underlying pigments, refer to the family heritage chart on page 159 to choose the dominant pigments. Normally people with **dark colored eyes** have hair with predominant **red undertones** and people with **light colored eyes** have predominant **yellow undertones** in their hair. This is a good guide to follow, however, will not always predict whether a client/guest has red or yellow undertones solely based on eye color. We always **recommend a strand test prior** to performing the haircolor service so both you and the client/guest can view the color results and make a decision whether the color formula needs to be adjusted.

Counterbalance Guideline

Hair with red undertones, use a green-base color

Hair with orange undertones, use a blue-base color

Hair with yellow undertones, use a purple-base color

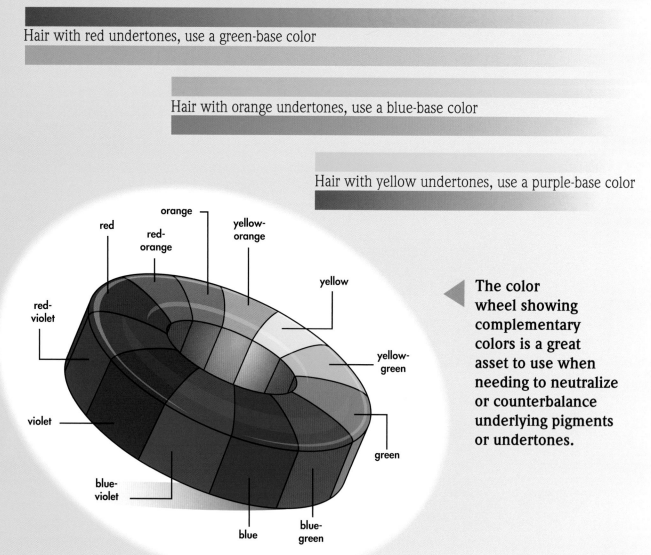

red
orange
red-orange
yellow-orange
yellow
red-violet
violet
yellow-green
green
blue-violet
blue
blue-green

The color wheel showing complementary colors is a great asset to use when needing to neutralize or counterbalance underlying pigments or undertones.

Alternative Haircolor Formulating ...

If applying a liquid color, *use the following basic mathematical equation to get the actual color level placed on the hair.*

Desired level x 2 - Natural level = Level used in color formula

Example:

1 **Desired (D) Level**
The client/guest's desired color is a level 7, **multiplied by 2,** equals 14.

$$7 \times 2 = 14$$

2 **Natural (N) Level**
Subtract the client/guest's natural level 5 from the doubled desired level 14; equals 9.

$$14 - 5 = 9$$

3 **Color Level Used in Color Formula**
Use the level 9 in a selected color series. Adjust formula by either moving up or down one to two levels depending on percentage of gray, porosity and/or undertones.

↓ 1 or 2 ↑

The mathematical equation of the **Desired level x 2 – Natural level = Level used in color formula** is based upon using **20 volumes** or 6 percent hydrogen peroxide in the color formulation. If the equation produces a level higher than 10, you may increase the volumes of hydrogen peroxide to be used.

- Use **25 volumes or 7.5%** of hydrogen peroxide to reach a **level 11.**

- Use **30 volumes or 9%** of hydrogen peroxide to reach a **level 12.**

- Any level higher than 12 would require a **double process** (lightener with toner) application.

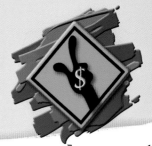

"Be sure to adjust color formula when increasing volumes/percentages of hydrogen peroxide to avoid creating orange or gold undertones."

Attend color manufacturer's classes and seminars for up-to-date information on the latest improvements and products available for professional haircolorists.

Hydrogen Peroxide Dilution ...

Liquid Hydrogen peroxide can be diluted to achieve the correct volume. **Dilution or reduction** is when a substance is weakened by adding another substance. **Distilled water** is used to dilute a high volume of hydrogen peroxide in order to obtain the correct volume needed. The hydrogen peroxide volume/percentage, whether it is 20, 30 or 40, plus the amount of distilled water, will produce the correct volume amount. Use the chart below when needing a 20 volume/percentage or less of hydrogen peroxide.

NOTE: If hydrogen peroxide is left unopened, the shelf life is usually about three years, but check with the product manufacturer.

Reduction (Dilution) of Stabilized Hydrogen Peroxide to Create the Desired Volume/Percentage of H_2O_2

Amount of 20 Volume H_2O_2	Distilled Water Ounces	Resulting Volume or Percentage
½ oz. of 20 volume	1 ½ oz. of water	5 volumes or 1 ½ %
1 oz. of 20 volume	1 oz. of water	10 volumes or 3 %
1½ oz. of 20 volume	½ oz. of water	15 volumes or 4 ½ %
2 oz. of 20 volume	None	20 volumes or 6 %
1 ¾ oz. of 25 volume	¼ oz. of water	20 volumes or 6 %
1 ½ oz. of 30 volume	½ oz. of water	20 volumes or 6 %
1 oz. of 40 volume	1 oz. of water	20 volumes or 6 %

* This chart is only used for clear H_2O_2, **not** the cream H_2O_2. Use a hydrometer to measure the diluted hydrogen peroxide.

Use this chart if the salon does not have the correct volume/percentage of hydrogen peroxide needed to create the color formula. Knowing there is an alternate way to create the required volume/percentage of H_2O_2 provides the haircolorist peace of mind.

To obtain the H_2O_2 volume amount, multiply the H_2O_2 percentage by 10 then divide by 3.

▶ $$H_2O_2 \% \times 10 \div 3$$

"Do not place hydrogen peroxide in a metal container – doing so may cause an adverse reaction. Mix hydrogen peroxide in a non-metallic (plastic or glass) bowl."

Volumes of Hydrogen Peroxide...

Reasons for using different volumes/percentages of hydrogen peroxide.

10 Volumes are used to **deposit pigment having no lightening action.** This is because it releases less oxygen gas, which is not enough strength to diffuse the natural melanin. Permanent haircolor may be mixed with 10 volumes hydrogen peroxide to deposit or enhance an already existing haircolor. Ten volumes of H_2O_2 mixed with lightener is used to slow down the development time to create equal processing time over entire head.

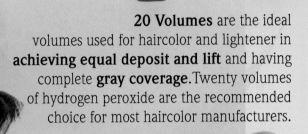

20 Volumes are the ideal volumes used for haircolor and lightener in **achieving equal deposit and lift** and having complete **gray coverage.** Twenty volumes of hydrogen peroxide are the recommended choice for most haircolor manufacturers.

30 Volumes are mixed with permanent haircolor and lightener to **achieve light and more vibrant colors on resistant hair.** The high volumes of hydrogen peroxide will increase the processing time. Stay with your client/guest and regularly perform development strand testing.

CAUTION: Prior to mixing lightener, read manufacturer's instructions to determine if any boosting or activating agents already exist in the packaged lightener. This will strengthen the development effects and possibly accelerate the color or lightener's processing time. Thirty volumes or higher of H_2O_2 are not recommended for anyone with a sensitive skin or scalp.

40 Volumes are used to create **ONLY high-lift haircolors** (one-step process) and are sometimes recommended for **off-the-scalp hair lightening services** depending on manufacturer. This high percentage of H_2O_2 developer **may cause hair damage** and is **not recommended for gray hair.** Always read the haircolor manufacturer's instructions before use.

Stages of Decolorization...

Seven Stages of Decolorization

STAGE 1
BLACK

STAGE 2
BROWN

STAGE 3
RED

STAGE 4
RED GOLD

STAGE 5
GOLD

STAGE 6
YELLOW

STAGE 7
PALE YELLOW

Hair lightener diffuses *or decolorizes the natural melanin or artificial pigment in the hair.* **Decolorizing** *is scattering or breaking up the pigments located in the cortex of the hair.* **The lightener is mixed with hydrogen peroxide** *along with other alkalizing agents to create the oxidation process. The scattering of melanin/pigment in the hair* **allows light reflection** *instead of absorption, which produces light shades of color. The longer the lightener remains on the hair, the more melanin/pigment will be diffused/scattered and the lighter the hair will become. As the pigment is diffusing, the hair changes in color, which is referred to as the* **seven stages of decolorization.**

"Hair that is naturally very dark reacts quickly to hair lightening. It oxidizes to the red-gold stage rapidly and then the oxidation process will suddenly decrease. Keep this in mind when formulating the desired color."

NOTE: The term bleaching has been replaced with more professional terms such as **decolorizing, decapping or color reduction.**

Steps of Color Separation ...

BLACK
(starting point)

10 Steps of Color Separation:

During the decolorization process, the underlying pigments in the hair are also diffused. As the hair is going through this process, the **undertones or underlying pigments** are revealed, whether the pigments are artificial (permanent color or lightener) or natural (exposure to sun). These **pigments will fall in between the seven stages of decolorization, BUT** are not always seen with the naked eye. This series of colors are referred to as the **10 steps of color separation.** During the hair service, be careful **not to decolorize further than the desired level** to preserve **some** of the underlying pigments. When color development is complete, the end color result will be a combination of the haircolor applied and the remaining underlying pigments.

BROWN — 1

DARK RED BROWN — 2

RED BROWN — 3

RED — 4

RED ORANGE — 5

DARK ORANGE — 6

LIGHT ORANGE — 7

GOLD — 8

YELLOW — 9

PALE YELLOW — 10

CAUTION: Avoid decolorizing or lightening past the pale yellow stage to prevent hair breakage. Do not lighten hair from a stage one to a stage seven ... susceptible to hair damage!

"Remember, the amount of pigment, density and porosity of the hair will influence the time of the decolorization process."

Not one head of hair is alike ... **all hair responds differently to haircolor.** This is the result of each individual's texture, porosity, elasticity and general overall condition of the hair as well as the client/guest's family heritage. Consider the following factors when formulating the color.

- **Fine texture hair** may process at a **darker color level** due to having a small diameter width. The general rule when formulating color for fine hair is to use one-half to one level lighter than desired level.

- **Coarse texture hair** may process at a **lighter color level** due to having a large diameter/width. The general rule when formulating color for this texture is to use one-half to one level darker.

- Hair with **unequal porosity accepts haircolor absorption unevenly.** Consider using a **color or conditioner filler** prior to color application when formulating the color mixture. This will equalize the hair porosity and/or add the missing primary color to obtain uniform color results. Strand test to determine which type of filler would provide the most successful color results.

- If a client/guest wants a lighter color than what was previously applied, first decolorize artificial pigment before recolorizing (applying new color). **You cannot lift color with color!**

Individual Considerations...

One of the biggest considerations a haircolorist may face while servicing client/guests is when the client/guest has natural brunette or very dark haircolor and it has been chemically altered by a permanent wave or relaxation. Hair with natural levels ranging from 1 to 3 has red undertones, which can impact various chemical services.

Below are a few suggestions to guide you in achieving successful color results.

- Client/guests with dark hair that has been treated with a thioglycolate relaxer or permanent wave could possibly reveal natural **red undertones**. A suggestion when formulating color for this particular client/guest is to consider either enhancing or neutralizing those red tones.

- **Brassy undertones** could emerge when trying to reach **more** than two levels of color in a single process application. For the most natural color results, process within two levels of the natural haircolor and use a 20 volume hydrogen peroxide.

- After approximately four to six weeks, the oxidative/permanent color fades, revealing **red undertones.** Use a color with a green base in your original color formula so that a soft, gold tone would appear as the color begins to fade.

  - **To prevent haircolor from fading,** apply an acid-balanced shampoo and conditioner to help close the cuticle and lock in the haircolor.

Avoid the following occurrences:
1) daily shampooing
2) swimming in chlorinated water
3) exposure to sunlight for long periods of time
4) using hair cleansing products that have a high pH

1

Individual Considerations ...

As with all chemical services, the hair becomes **susceptible to dryness and/or damage** due to the use of alkalizing agents needed to perform the chemical services. There are some **preventative solutions** that could be utilized to prevent overprocessing and minimize hair damage. It is always recommended to postpone a chemical service if hair breakage already exists to avoid further damage.

- It is recommended to **wait a minimum of one week after a chemical relaxing service** before applying haircolor.

- Use **low volumes of hydrogen peroxide** when coloring hair that has been chemically relaxed.

- A **double process service is not recommended** on hair that has been chemically relaxed due to the two-step process of lightening and toning.

- Newly **permanent waved hair should be strand tested** prior to getting a **double process service.** The chemicals used in a permanent wave can dry or damage the hair, therefore a series of reconstructor treatments might have to be recommended before another chemical service is applied.

- Previous color treatments can affect how the hair responds to a **new and different haircolor.** Do not reapply haircolor over previously colored hair without taking a strand test – color on color can create a build-up on the hair, especially porous areas of hair.

- When performing a retouch and the **remaining hair has faded and needs to be refreshed,** dilute your color mixture with conditioner or shampoo (known as soap cap) and apply to the mid-strands and hair ends during the last 5 to 10 minutes of development time – check manufacturer's directions.

Individual Considerations ...

Another area of concern is **progressive haircoloring,** which gradually develops the haircolor through repeated applications. **Metallic salts** are an ingredient used in some home-haircoloring kits, especially men's haircoloring, which leaves a **metal coating on the hair.** This may effect and interfere with product absorption of other chemical services. The type of metal used determines the color outcome; for example, copper will produce a red color or lead will create a brown to black color. If the client/guest is requesting other chemical services, the potential of hair discoloration, severe breakage or irregular curl patterns can occur. Whenever the professional is unsure of color used on the client/guest's hair, **perform a metallic salt test.** Cut a ½ inch (1.25 cm) of hair from an inconspicuous area on the head and follow the procedure below.

Test for Metallic Salts on the Hair:

- Mix one ounce 20 volume hydrogen peroxide with 20 drops of 28 percent ammonia in glass container.

- Place approximately 20 hair strands into a container and soak for 30 minutes.

- **If no metallic salts are present,** hair will lighten slightly. Hair **may receive other chemical services.**

- Hair with a lead coating will lighten quickly.

- Hair with a silver coating has no reaction within the 30 minutes.

- Hair with a copper coating will break apart; the solution will boil and produce an unpleasant odor.

CAUTION: Hair with a lead, silver or copper coating **CANNOT** receive any chemical services. The hair affected by the metals must either be cut off or some manufacturers will offer a prepared solution to remove the metals from the hair. Check with the local beauty distributor.

Dimensional Haircoloring...

Dimensional haircoloring techniques are the placement of **highlights, lowlights or various base shapes** on selected pieces or subsections of hair. The dimensional techniques may cover either a full or partial area of the head. Dimensional techniques stimulate the imagination by allowing the haircolorist to **create arrangements of two or more colors** anywhere on the head. The concept behind dimensional haircoloring applies the theory that **light colors bring out** or add brightness and **dark colors recede** or create depth in a hairdesign. The special effects provide contrast, illusion of depth, light reflection and/or textures on the hair, making it a popular haircoloring service.

Highlighting and lowlighting is achieved through a **foiling technique,** which is placing a small piece of foil under a selected subsection of hair.

NOTE: The word **"highlighting"** is a general term that means selected pieces of hair, which are lightened or lifted above the client/guest's existing color level.

SLICING

WEAVING

The **foiling technique** is performed by either **weaving or slicing** subsections of hair. **To highlight hair,** a lightener or high-lift oxidative color is placed on the selected hair strands. **For the client/guest wanting lowlights,** a low-level haircolor is applied on the selected hair strands. The weave or sliced hair is enclosed in the foil by folding the foil in half and turning each side in toward the center to create a packet. Processing is achieved by oxidation of color or lightener, body heat or an external heat source (hooded dryer or accelerator machine). Positioning client/guest under an external heat source will increase the development time and/or lightening action. Check with haircolor/lightener manufacturer's directions before using any type of external heat for processing.

Dimensional Haircoloring...

Two Foiling Techniques

The size of the subsections and the amount of hair weaved or sliced is determined by the desired end color result and hairdesign. **Large subsections with a heavy weave or slice** creates a channeled and bolder appearance of color. **Small subsections with a light weave or slice** provides a blended color effect. If client/guest has curly hair, it is recommended to apply a medium to heavy weave for optimal visual color results. Refer to Chapter 7 for several foiling technique procedures.

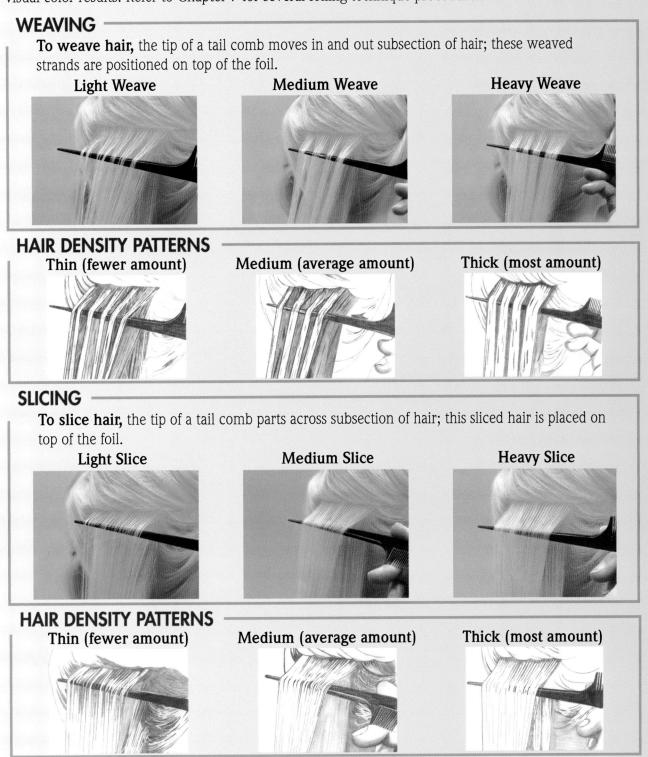

WEAVING

To weave hair, the tip of a tail comb moves in and out subsection of hair; these weaved strands are positioned on top of the foil.

| Light Weave | Medium Weave | Heavy Weave |

HAIR DENSITY PATTERNS

| Thin (fewer amount) | Medium (average amount) | Thick (most amount) |

SLICING

To slice hair, the tip of a tail comb parts across subsection of hair; this sliced hair is placed on top of the foil.

| Light Slice | Medium Slice | Heavy Slice |

HAIR DENSITY PATTERNS

| Thin (fewer amount) | Medium (average amount) | Thick (most amount) |

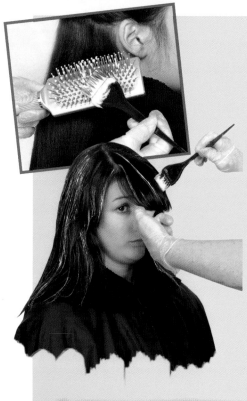

Free hand, free form or surface painting is a technique where the professional is in control of the tool and **manually places haircolor or lightener on the hair surface.** You are the artist ... paint, comb or brush color or lightener on the surface of clean, dry or damp hair following the client/guest's hairdesign. **Both highlights and lowlights** can be achieved using this technique. The color or lightener can also be placed on the hair by dividing the hair into sections and applying on each section (refer to Chapter 7 for procedure). **Baliage** is another term used for this technique, which is a **French term meaning, "strands of color."**

An alternative to free hand painting is the **"shoe-shine" or "sun-kissed" method,** which is accomplished by placing **lightener on a sheet of foil,** covering one side only. The professional will hold the foil and lightly press against the hair surface, pull foil off hair and press again, continuing to move around the hairdesign, repeating the technique. The end result is very natural-looking. There are endless possibilities using the free hand painting techniques.

The **cap and hook method** is pulling clean, dry hair through a perforated plastic or latex cap using a crochet hook. Another term used for this technique is **frosting**. The length of hair recommended for this method is 4 inches (10.16 cm) or shorter. The amount of hair pulled through each hole, or if every hole is used, depends upon hair density and desired color result. If a **subtle color effect** is desired, pull less hair from **every other hole.** If client/guest wants a **dramatic color finish,** use **every hole** and pull more hair from each hole. Once the selected hair is pulled, comb through hair to remove any tangles and check for consistency on hair amount pulled over entire head. Highlights or lowlights may be achieved by placing either a lightener or haircolor on the hair. When development time is complete, do not remove cap, rinse product from hair and apply shampoo, then remove cap (shampoo allows easy removal of cap) and complete entire head with cleansing and conditioning. Using the cap and hook technique is a time-saver, but does not always create the accuracy that can be achieved with foils.

Another color effect called **tipping** may also be created by using either the free hand painting or cap and hook technique – being careful to place color or lightener **ONLY on the hair ends.** The ends of hair are secured so as not to come in contact with previously colored hair or the mid-strand to scalp portion of hair.

Dimensional Haircoloring...

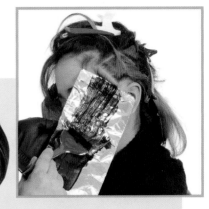

The **zonal technique** consists of **sectioned areas or patterns** on the head where two or more colors are placed. The patterns, whether they are in the **nape, crown, fringe, perimeter or front hairline,** are separated from the rest of the hair – the sectioned hair receives a color or lightener and the rest of the hair gets a different color or lightener. More than one pattern can be placed on the head at one time. Zonal haircoloring creates contrasting color results, provides a focal point and derives interest within its color design. The results can range from bold and striking to mild and subtle, depending on the client/guest's wishes.

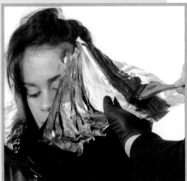

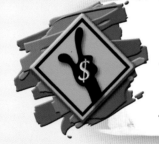

To help increase your service ticket, encourage dimensional haircoloring services to your existing color client/guests! Be your own source of advertisement by having highlights and/ or lowlights in your own hair. As an introductory dimensional haircoloring service to your client/guest, offer to place a few face-framing highlights in his or her hair.

An alternative to the zonal technique is creating specific *base shape patterns* within the hairdesign. The base shapes are various **geometric shapes** subsectioned in the hair, creating contrasting color results. Base shapes such as **triangles, circles and rectangles (channeling)** are some of the shapes used for creative color designing, but other shapes can be used; the possibilities are endless when you use your imagination.

With both these techniques, semi-, demi-, permanent haircolor or lightener may be used to achieve optimal results.

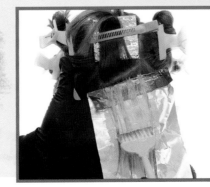

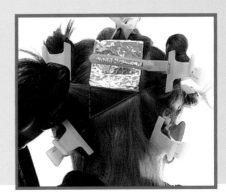

Lightener with Toner ...

If a client/guest requests a blonde haircolor, but his or her natural color level is too dark and the haircolorist is unable to reach the desired blonde color using a permanent (oxidative) color, the next recommendation is to offer the double process service. **The double process service is when a lightener and toner are applied,** which involves two applications to reach the end color result.

In the first application, hair is decolorized or pre-lightened to a desired level using lightener (bleach). **In the second application, hair is recolorized** by applying haircolor, either semi-, demi- or permanent color to reach the desired blonde shade. Refer to Chapter 6 to view the step-by-step double process procedure.

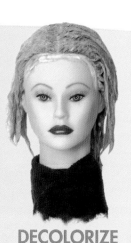
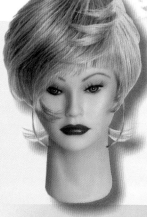

DECOLORIZE   **RECOLORIZE**

Important Reminders:

- **Development strand testing is necessary** in both the pre-lightening and toning phase of this procedure. The strand test will determine when the hair has reached the level of lightness while decolorizing, and the desired blonde color when recolorizing.

- **Small 1/8 inch (0.3 cm) partings are required** in order to have consistent lightener absorption.

- When **applying lightener, keep ½ to 1 inch (1.25 cm to 2.5 cm) away from scalp and hair ends** because both areas process quicker. The scalp area is affected by body heat and the hair ends are generally porous.

- Once hair has **reached 50 percent of the desired level** (strand test to check level), take **1/8 inch (0.3 cm) partings** and apply lightener to the scalp and hair ends. Process hair until full desired level has been achieved – again, strand test to determine the full level. Rinse, shampoo, lightly condition and towel blot hair.

- The hair is resectioned for recolorizing service.

- Non-oxidative or oxidative color is applied from scalp to hair ends, **taking ¼ inch (0.6 cm) partings.**

- **Development strand test** is taken to decide when color has fully absorbed and processing is complete. Rinse, shampoo and condition (to close cuticle) hair.

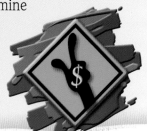

- For a retouch double process, **apply lightener at new growth ONLY ... avoid overlapping lightener onto previously lightened hair** to prevent hair damage and breakage.

In order for double process (lightened) hair to appear healthy, conditioning treatments are essential. Recommend to the client/guest weekly conditioning treatment services that consist of both protein and moisturizing ingredients.

Perform Strand Testing ...

RA

8

Step Eight
Perform a preliminary strand test

Preliminary strand testing is taking a small subsection of hair and **applying the pre-determined color formula on the hair.** *Process, rinse and dry hair; then the client/guest and you are able to view the color results prior to placing over entire head. This will give an exact development time (porosity), plus provide a great preview of the color results.*

Advantages of preliminary strand testing:

- Show actual color formula results prior to placing over entire head

- Determine the exact processing time

- Demonstrate the reaction of the hair to decide if any special treatments (fillers) are needed to assist with color absorption

- Detect residues from previous haircolor applications (metallic or compound dyes)

Perform Strand Testing ...

Development/Processing strand testing is taking a small subsection of hair **during processing to view the color or lightener results.** It will determine if color is properly developed/processed and if it has absorbed evenly along the hair strand. For hair lightening, it will show the accurate stage of decolorization. The subsection of hair is wiped free of color or lightener product and viewed in natural light to make an accurate determination if color or stage of decolorization is developed.

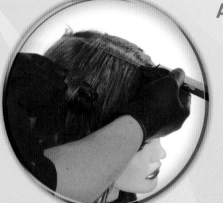

Advantages of development/processing strand testing:

○ Provides an accurate development time

○ Able to view for equal color or lightener absorption

○ Shows concise stage of development or decolorization

9 Step Nine

Complete a client/ guest record card (written or electronic) of the color service.

RETAIL • RE-BOOK • REFERRAL

It is important to record the results of all color services, either digitally or written on an actual client/guest card, so that successful formulations can be reproduced and/or any problems can be avoided for future services. Make sure all pertinent information is recorded for future appointments to eliminate any displeased client/guests. To keep safe, reliable and confidential client/guest cards, it is recommended to electronically produce and record all client/guest information.

At the conclusion of the service, recommend a series of products (shampoo, conditioner, etc.) for **home-care use** in order to maintain the condition of the hair and longevity of the haircolor until returning to the salon. This action should not be overlooked because the client/guest is your source of advertisement and we want him or her to be happy with the service and return to the salon.

Client/Guest Haircolor Level: Natural ___ Desired ___ Percentage of Gray_____
Haircolor Formulation: _____
Timing: _____
First Time Color Results: _____
Retouch Color Formulation: _____
Retouch Results: _____
Service Date with Cost: _____

DATE	SERVICE/TREATMENT-Formula/Product/Procedure	REMARKS/CHANGES

CLIENT/GUEST RECORD CARD

Name _Jane Doe_ Date _3/9/12_ Cosmetologist _Sally_ License # _78291_

Address _123 First Street_ Hair Condition: Normal _X_Dry __ Breakage __ Scalp Condition: Normal_X_Dry __ Oily __

Home Phone _____ Work _____ Mobile _____ Texture: Fine __ Medium __ Coarse _X_ Type of Hair: Straight_X_Wavy __ Curly __

Email Address _www.janedoe.com_ Density: Thick __ Medium_X_Thin __

Birthdate (month/day)_7/6_ Occupation _housewife_ Porosity: Resistant __ Normal _X_Severe __ Irregular __

First Visit Date _7/2/81_ Elasticity: Average_X_Low __ Length: Short __ Medium __ Long_X_

Patch Test Administered: Date/Initials Examined: Date/Initials

Check all that apply: Results: Positive __ Negative _X_ _9/14/SW_

Medications __ Allergies __ What attracted you to our salon? Friend_X_ Location __ Advertisement __

Personal Hair-Care Products: Shampoo_X_Conditioner __ Hairspray __ Gel __Other __ REMARKS _____

Professional Haircoloring: Temporary __ Semi-Permanent _X_Demi-Permanent __

Permanent __ Lightener __ Home Haircolor __

I receive the following chemical services: Color_X_Perm __ Lightening __ Relaxer__

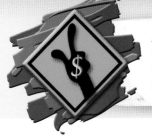

Always ask a returning client/guest about his or her haircolor quality since the last salon visit. Suggest new ideas to enhance color appearance. This not only improves your customer/guest service skills, but may increase your total service ticket.

Nine Steps of Haircoloring

The main areas of the haircoloring service are broken down into **nine major steps** for the professional to follow. Use these nine steps as your guide to make sure every part is successfully completed – this will result in a thorough color service.

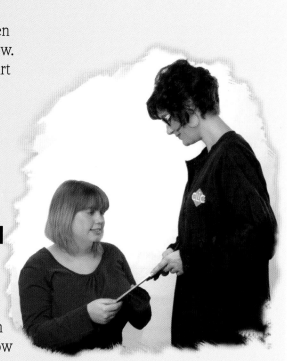

STEP ONE

CONDUCT A CLIENT/GUEST CONSULTATION

The **consultation**, referred to as **"chair talk,"** is the first essential step of the haircoloring service. This is the cosmetologists' opportunity to ask questions and establish a relationship with the client/guest in order to get to know his or her hair-care needs and desired haircolor.

STEP TWO

PERFORM A PREDISPOSITION (PATCH) TEST

Allergy is a **hypersensitivity response** to a normally harmless substance to which the body reacts. It is an antigen-antibody disorder, reaction or extreme sensitivity to chemicals, drugs, foods, animals and other substances.

Predisposition or patch test is applying a small amount of the haircolor mixture on the skin to check for skin sensitivity of products/chemicals.

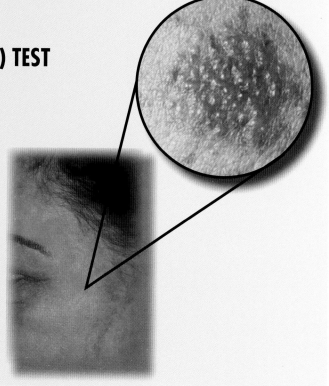

STEP THREE

DETERMINE THE CLIENT/GUEST'S NATURAL OR BASE HAIRCOLOR LEVEL

An individual's natural or base haircolor is derived from the **melanocyte cells located in the cortex layer** of the hair. **Natural haircolor** basically ranges in shades from **black, brown, red and blonde.** The color is broken down into levels and each level is given a number from 1 to 10.

Level or value is determining the **degree of lightness or darkness of a color** depending on how much light is reflected or absorbed.

For Example:

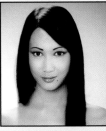

Number 1
Black

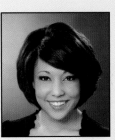

Number 5
Medium Brown

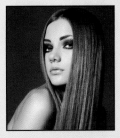

Number 7
Medium Blonde

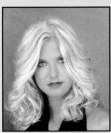

Number 10
Lightest Blonde

Haircolor Families or Series

Most professional haircolor manufacturers will display their haircolors on hair swatches placed in a **chart or binder.** Every manufacturer will design and identify its haircolors differently ... the level numbering and color identification will vary.

N – Neutral or Natural Series
A – Ash Series
G – Gold Series
R – Red Series
B – Beige Series
HL – High-Lift Blonde Series

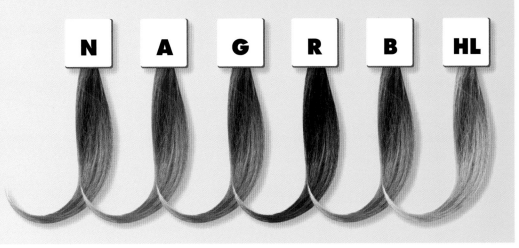

STEP FOUR

DETERMINE THE CLIENT/GUEST'S DESIRED COLOR SHADE/LEVEL

The client/guest will use a haircolor chart to select the desired level and color of his or her liking.

NATURAL/NEUTRAL is a blend of all **three primary colors, but in unequal proportions,** resulting in more natural shades. This series is available in **10 levels –** level 1 (blue black) to level 10 (lightest blonde).

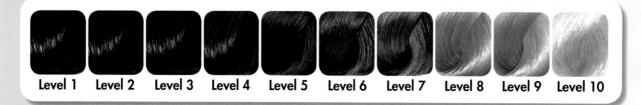

| Level 1 | Level 2 | Level 3 | Level 4 | Level 5 | Level 6 | Level 7 | Level 8 | Level 9 | Level 10 |

ASH is **unequal mixtures of blue and violet base shades** with no primary yellow, which are arranged in **levels of 4 to 10.**

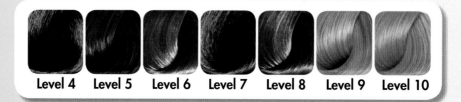

| Level 4 | Level 5 | Level 6 | Level 7 | Level 8 | Level 9 | Level 10 |

GOLD colors consist of **red and yellow** with yellow being the predominant tone. This family of color is available in **levels 4 to 10**, providing **soft golden shades.**

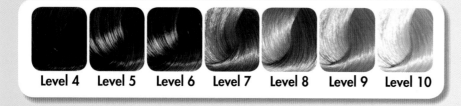

| Level 4 | Level 5 | Level 6 | Level 7 | Level 8 | Level 9 | Level 10 |

RED series has varying red colors with either a **base of yellow (warm) or a base of violet (cool).** The red series ranges from **levels 4 to 8** and generally falls under the red-violet or red-orange category.

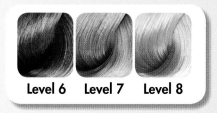

Level 4   Level 5   Level 6   Level 7   Level 8

BEIGE is a **blend of red, yellow and blue** with less intensity than the natural/neutral family. The beige family is available in **levels 6 to 8.**

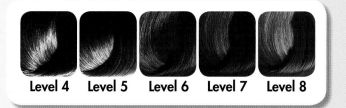

Level 6   Level 7   Level 8

BLONDE consists of **unequal proportions of red, yellow and blue with a high concentration of yellow.** The blonde series ranges from **level 7 to 10 or higher** depending on manufacturer.

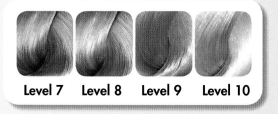

Level 7   Level 8   Level 9   Level 10

HIGH-LIFT BLONDES include the families of ash, beige, gold and natural.

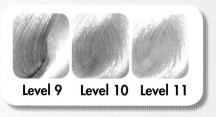

Level 9   Level 10   Level 11

STEP FIVE

DETERMINE THE AMOUNT OF WHITE/GRAY HAIR

Gray hair is the result of a **gradual or slowing down of melanin** production in the cortex layer of the hair. Generally, most client/guests will have a percentage of gray hair; meaning a combination of pigmented (gray) hair and non-pigmented (white) hair, referred to as "salt and pepper" hair.

When hair has a **total absence of pigment** – no eumelanin or pheomelanin, it is referred to as **white hair.**

Gray Hair Percentage

Level System	25 Percent – more gray hair, less white hair	50 Percent – an equal mixture of gray and white hair	75 Percent – less gray hair, more white hair
LIGHT	25%	50%	75%
MEDIUM	25%	50%	75%
DARK	25%	50%	75%

STEP SIX

DETERMINE COLOR SATURATION/REFLECTION

Color saturation works in conjunction with color intensity. It is a combination of pigment concentration and light reflection that results in a multitude of colors. Permanent oxidative colors will also **contain alkalizing agents** such as ammonia to assist in color saturation and/or reflection.

The **greater amount** of alkalizing agents in the color, **more color reflection** is achieved with **less color saturation** … hence, **high levels of color** are produced. The **less amount** of alkalizing agents in the color, **the less color reflection** is achieved with **more color saturation;** therefore, **low levels of color** are produced.

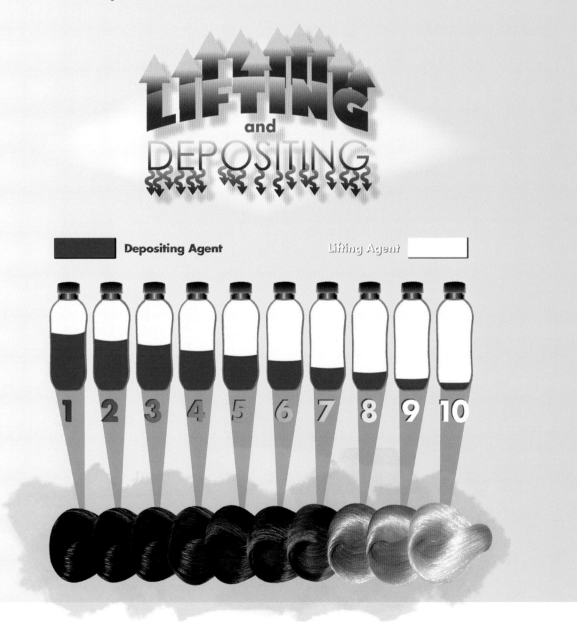

Depositing Agent   Lifting Agent

1 2 3 4 5 6 7 8 9 10

Nine Steps of Haircoloring

STEP SEVEN

CREATE THE COLOR FORMULA

Color formulating is a standard four-part approach when determining the actual color formula/mixture used on the client/guest's hair.

1. Determine client/guest's natural or base level from the color manufacturer's color chart using the natural series.

2. Choose the client/guest's desired color, which includes the color's level, family and tonality of color.

3. If present, determine percentage of gray – use salt (white hair) and pepper (pigmented hair) as your guide.

4. Decide the volumes/percentages of hydrogen peroxide used to create the color formula.

  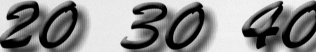 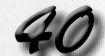

Ten Volumes/3% H_2O_2	Twenty Volumes/6% H_2O_2	Thirty Volumes/9% H_2O_2	Forty Volumes/12% H_2O_2
For going darker than natural/base level	For depositing at base level	For going two levels lighter than natural/base level	Going three levels lighter than base level
Use for toning pre-lightened hair	Going one level lighter than natural/base level	Going three levels lighter using an intensifier (check manufacturer's directions)	Going four levels lighter using an intensifier (chek manufacturer's directions)
	For optimum gray coverage		

STEP EIGHT

PREFORM A PRELIMINARY STRAND TEST

Preliminary strand testing is taking a small subsection of hair and **applying the pre-determined color formula on the hair.** This will give an exact development time (porosity), plus provide a great preview of the color results.

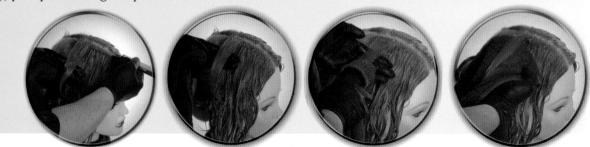

Nine Steps of Haircoloring

STEP NINE

COMPLETE A CLIENT/GUEST RECORD CARD
(WRITTEN OR ELECTRONIC) OF THE COLOR SERVICE

It is important to record the results of all color services either digitally or written on an actual client/guest card, so that successful formulations can be reproduced and/or any problems can be avoided for future services. Make sure all pertinent information is recorded for future appointments to eliminate any displeased client/guests. To keep safe, reliable and confidential client/guest cards, it is recommended to electronically produce and record all client/guest information.

CLIENT/GUEST RECORD CARD

Name _____ Date _____ Cosmetologist _____ License # _____
Address _____ Hair Condition: Normal __ Dry __ Breakage __ Scalp Condition: Normal __ Dry __ Oily __
Home Phone _____ Work _____ Mobile _____ Texture: Fine ___ Medium __ Coarse __ Type of Hair: Straight __ Wavy __ Curly __
Email Address _____ Density: Thick __ Medium __ Thin __
Birthdate (month/day) _____ Occupation _____ Porosity: Resistant __ Normal __ Severe __ Irregular __
First Visit Date _____ Elasticity: Average __ Low __ Length: Short __ Medium __ Long __
Patch Test Administered: Date/Initials Examined: Date/Initials
Check All that Apply: Results: Positive __ Negative __
Medications __ Allergies __ What attracted you to our salon? Friend __ Location __ Advertisement __
Personal Haircare Products: Shampoo __ Conditioner __ Hairspray __ Gel __Other __ REMARKS _____
Professional Haircoloring: Temporary __ Semi-Permanent __ Demi-Permanent __
Permanent __ Lightener __ Home Haircolor __
I Receive the Following Chemical Services: Color __ Perm __ Lightening __ Relaxer __

Client/Guest Haircolor Level: Natural ___ Desired ___ Percent__
Haircolor Formulation: _____
Timing: _____
First Time Color Results: _____
Retouch Color Formulation: _____
Retouch Results: _____
Service Date with Cost: _____

DATE	SERVICE/TREATMENT-Formula/Product/Procedure	REMARKS/CHANGES

CLIENT/GUEST RECORD CARD

Name _Jane Doe_ Date _3/9/12_ Cosmetologist _Sally_ License # _78291_
Address _123 First Street_ Hair Condition: Normal __ Dry X Breakage __ Scalp Condition: Normal X Dry __ Oily __
Home Phone _____ Work _____ Mobile _____ Texture: Fine ___ Medium __ Coarse X Type of Hair: Straight X Wavy __ Curly __
Email Address _www.janedoe.com_ Density: Thick __ Medium __ Thin X
Birthdate (month/day) _7/6_ Occupation _housewife_ Porosity: Resistant __ Normal X Severe __ Irregular __
First Visit Date _7/2/81_ Elasticity: Average X Low __ Length: Short __ Medium __ Long X
Patch Test Administered: Date/Initials Examined: Date/Initials
Check all that apply: Results: Positive __ Negative X _9/14/SW_
Medications __ Allergies __ What attracted you to our salon? Friend X Location __ Advertisement __
Personal Hair-Care Products: Shampoo X Conditioner __ Hairspray __ Gel __Other __ REMARKS _____
Professional Haircoloring: Temporary __ Semi-Permanent X Demi-Permanent __ _____
Permanent __ Lightener __ Home Haircolor __
I receive the following chemical services: Color X Perm __ Lightening __ Relaxer __

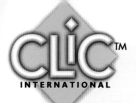

A.	Cap and Hook Method
B.	Client/Guest Record Card
C.	Color Saturation
D.	Consultation
E.	Decolorizing
F.	Double Process
G.	Free Form Painting
H.	Gray Hair
I.	Highlighting
J.	High Numbers
K.	Letters
L.	Level
M.	Lowlighting
N.	Negative Patch Test
O.	Neutral or Natural Series
P.	Preliminary Strand Testing
Q.	Pre-softening
R.	Release Statement
S.	Sulfer
T.	10 Volume H$_2$O$_2$

FILL-IN-THE-BLANKS

1. _____ consists of colors ranging from a level 1 to 10 and has a blend of all three primary colors.

2. _____ is used for going darker than natural level and for toning pre-lightened hair.

3. _____ is applying lightener or a high-lift oxidative color on selected hair strands placed on a piece of foil.

4. _____ referred to as "chair talk," is the first essential step of the haircoloring service.

5. _____ indicates there is no sensitivity to the haircolor product.

6. _____ is the result of a gradual or slowing down of melanin production in the cortex.

7. _____ is scattering or breaking up the pigments located in the cortex of the hair.

8. _____ is the degree of lightness or darkness of a color.

9. _____ identify the series or families of color on the haircolor swatch chart.

10. _____ is filled out before and after a haircoloring service.

11. _____ is placing a product on resistant areas of the hair to initiate the process of opening the cuticle scales.

12. _____ is a form affirming the client/guest was advised of the potential risks that could result during the chemical procedure.

13. _____ pigmentation occurs with people that have light eyes.

14. _____ is when the color or lightener is placed on the hair surface manually by the professional.

15. _____ is the application of a lightener and toner in two separate steps.

16. _____ indicate light levels of color.

17. _____ is applying a low-level haircolor on selected hair strands placed on a piece of foil.

18. _____ is a combination of pigment concentration and light reflection that results in a multitude of colors.

19. _____ is applying a pre-determined color formula on a small subsection of hair to preview color results.

20. _____ is pulling clean, dry hair through a perforated plastic or latex cap using a crochet hook.

STUDENT'S NAME   DATE   GRADE

allergy   darker
      lighter
permanent
        predisposition
    retouch
       temporary

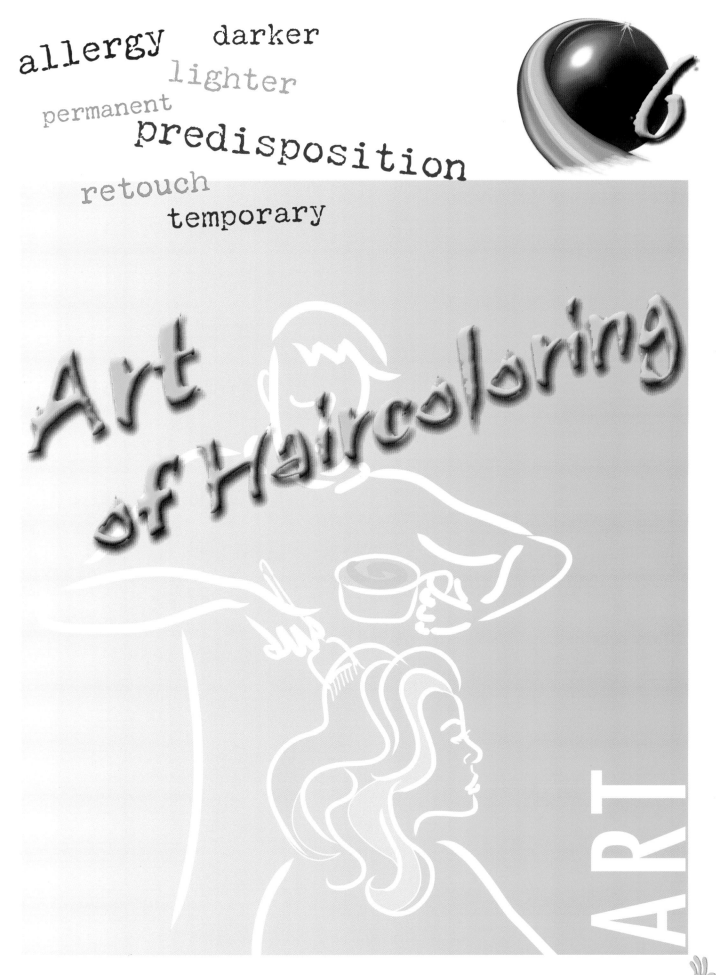

Art of Haircoloring

ART

Predisposition or Patch Test

OBJECTIVE

To perform and determine if the client/ guest has a sensitivity/allergy to an aniline derivative haircolor. This ingredient may be in semi-permanent, demi-permanent and permanent haircolors.

According to the U.S. Food, Drug Cosmetic Act, this test must be performed 24-48 hours prior to the haircolor service.

TOOLS & MATERIALS

- Cloth and disposable towels
- Gloves
- Chemical apron
- Measuring cup
- Cotton or cotton-tipped applicators
- Haircolor product
- Hydrogen peroxide
- Sectioning clips
- Color bowl and brush
- Client/guest record card
- Skin cleanser

PROCEDURE

"The client/guest consultation is an important part of your professional service. Be sure to complete this step prior to each client/guest service you provide. Your successful retail sales and customer satisfaction rates depend upon it!"

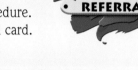
RETAIL • RE-BOOK • REFERRAL

1. Cosmetologist sanitizes hands and station.
2. Set out service tools and materials.
3. Follow procedure as shown and manufacturer's instructions.
4. Follow standard cleanup procedure.
5. Document client/guest record card.

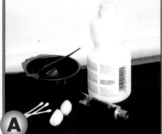

A. Table set up with required tools and materials.

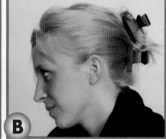

B. Select the area to be tested, if using **behind ear**, clip hair back from hairline and place towel over shoulder.

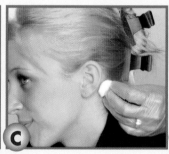

C. Clean behind ear, along hairline with warm water and cleanser. Dry area.

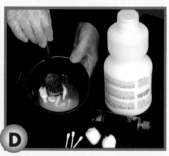

D. Mix a small amount of haircolor with hydrogen peroxide following manufacturer's instructions. Client/guest's actual or a similar color mixture is used.

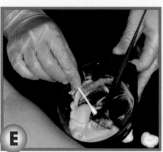

E. Using a cotton-tipped applicator, immerse into color mixture.

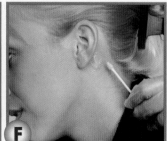

F. Apply a small amount of color mixture to cleansed area behind ear.

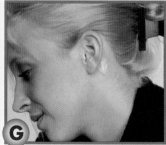

G. Let dry. **Do not remove or disturb the color for 24 to 48 hours.**

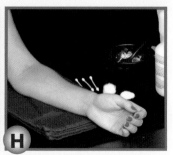

H. If testing on **inner fold of elbow**, rest arm on a small towel.

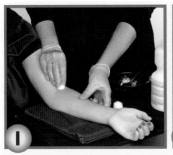

I Clean a small area on inner fold of elbow with warm water and cleanser. Dry area.

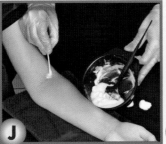

J Use a cotton-tipped applicator and apply small amount of color mixture to inner fold area of elbow.

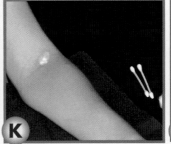

K Let dry. **Do not remove or disturb the color for 24 to 48 hours.**

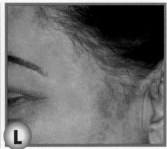

L **If a positive reaction occurs** (indicating redness, swelling or itching), remove color from area and report to cosmetologist **– Do not perform haircoloring service.**

M No symptoms will indicate a negative reaction, proceed with haircolor service.

NOTE: Severe allergic reactions show up as trouble breathing, swallowing and thickness of tongue or blistering of skin. If symptoms for a positive reaction are severe, call a medical care professional immediately.

Preliminary and Development/ Processing Strand Testing

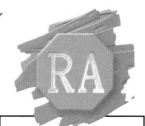

OBJECTIVE

Preliminary strand testing is applying the desired color formula to a subsection of hair in order to preview color results prior to color service. **Development/processing strand testing** involves removing color from a small subsection of hair to determine absorption of color and if processing is complete.

Check with your local regulatory agency to see if the predisposition test is required 24-48 hours prior to the haircolor service.

TOOLS & MATERIALS

- Cloth and disposable towels
- Measuring cup
- Hydrogen peroxide
- Sectioning clips
- Color chart

- Airformer
- Color bowl and brush
- Haircolor product
- Neck strip and cape/robe
- Hydrometer

- Timer
- Haircoloring foils
- Chemical apron
- Water bottle
- Shampoo and conditioner

- Gloves
- Applicator bottle
- Coloring combs
- Client/guest record card

PROCEDURE

"The client/guest consultation is an important part of your professional service. Be sure to complete this step prior to each client/guest service you provide. Your successful retail sales and customer satisfaction rates depend upon it!"

1. Cosmetologist sanitizes hands and station.
2. Set out service tools and materials.
3. Drape client/guest in preparation for chemical service.
4. Perform scalp and hair analysis.
5. Follow procedure as shown and manufacturer's instructions.

6. Follow standard cleanup procedure.
7. Document client/guest record card.

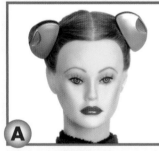

A Divide clean, dry hair into four sections.

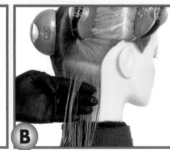

B Select a subsection of hair in a discreet location of head, preferably the most resistant, darkest or grayest area.

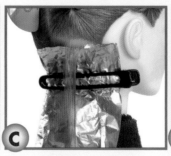

C Desired amount of hair used for subsection is **½ to 1 inch (1.25 to 2.5 cm)**. Place one foil under the selected hair to protect the remaining hair not being tested.

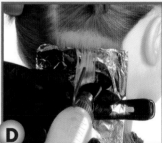

D Prepare a small amount of the desired color formula in bowl or applicator bottle. Apply color directly on the clean, dry hair.

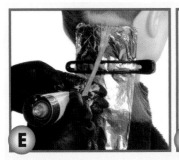

E Cover entire subsection of hair for even color absorption.

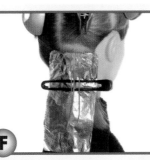

F Process color following manufacturer's instructions.

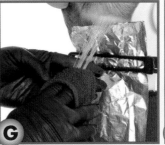

G When processing is complete, wipe color from hair using a cloth towel.

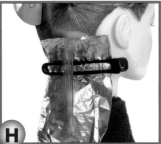

H The cosmetologist and client/guest observe the color results under natural light. Discuss with the client/guest and modify if necessary or proceed with haircolor service.

Development/Processing Strand Testing:

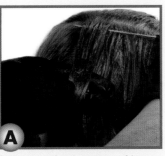

A Part a small subsection of hair from a most resistant, dark or gray area of the head.

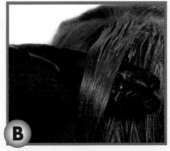

B Place section of hair on top of fingers to separate from the hair that is still processing.

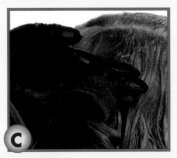

C Wipe color from hair using a cloth towel.

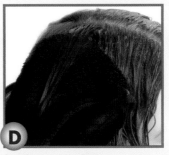

D Observe color results to determine if development/processing is complete or if more time is needed.

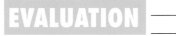

EVALUATION _____

_____

GRADE _____ STUDENT'S NAME _____ ID# _____

Temporary Haircolor

OBJECTIVE

To introduce haircolor that adds a slight color change to the hair. **NOTE:** Since temporary haircolor covers the cuticle layer of the hair, it will only last until the next hair cleansing, unless hair is extremely porous.

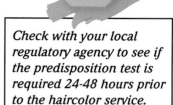

Check with your local regulatory agency to see if the predisposition test is required 24-48 hours prior to the haircolor service.

Before

TOOLS & MATERIALS

- Cloth and disposable towels
- Gloves
- Chemical apron
- Neck strip and cape/robe
- Timer
- Color chart
- Color bowl and brush
- Measuring cup
- Applicator bottle
- Styling brushes
- Shampoo and conditioner
- Sectioning clips
- Coloring combs
- Temporary color product
- Thermal tools
- Color stain remover
- Liquid styling tools
- Client/guest record card

PROCEDURE

"The client/guest consultation is an important part of your professional service. Be sure to complete this step prior to each client/guest service you provide. Your successful retail sales and customer satisfaction rates depend upon it!"

RETAIL RE-BOOK REFERRAL

1. Cosmetologist sanitizes hands and station.
2. Set out service tools and materials.
3. Drape client/guest in preparation for chemical service.
4. Perform scalp and hair analysis along with preliminary strand testing.
5. Follow procedure as shown and manufacturer's instructions.
6. Follow standard cleanup procedure.
7. Document client/guest record card.

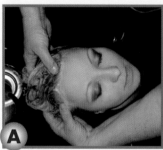

A Lightly cleanse hair and scalp. **DO NOT** manipulate to avoid scalp sensitivity.

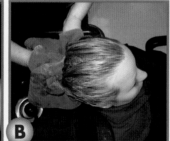

B Towel-dry hair, absorbing any excess water.

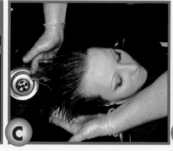

C Depending on color viscosity (thickness), this type of color can be applied while client/guest is still reclined in shampoo bowl.

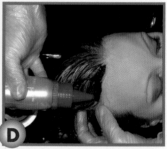

D Apply color along hairline using fingers of the opposite hand to guide color along hair strands.

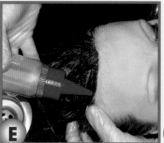

E Spread color into hair using your thumb and fingers.

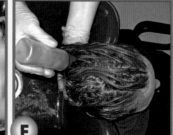

F Continue applying color moving back toward occipital portion of head.

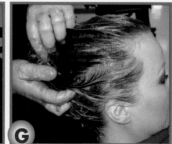

G Guide color along hair strands to cover the hair at back of head.

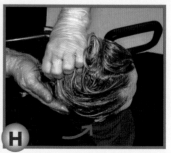

H Slightly turn client/guest's head to apply a generous amount of color to hair behind the ear.

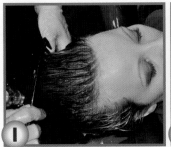

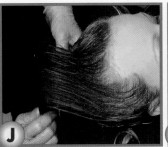

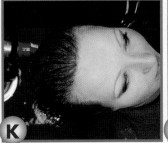

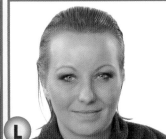

I Once color is applied, check manufacturer's instructions if color is required to be combed through for even distribution and absorption.

J Continue to comb color through hair for complete coverage.

K Follow manufacturer's instructions for processing and if the color **is or is not** rinsed and shampooed from hair.

L Proceed with finished design.

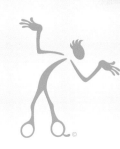

M Completed temporary haircolor.

"Every haircolor product varies in its chemical components, viscosities and placement ... please always read your manufacturer's instructions before proceeding with color service."

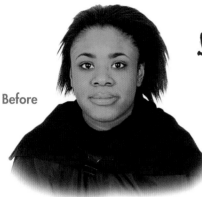

Before

Semi-Permanent Haircolor

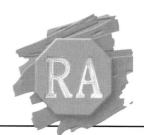

RA

Check with your local regulatory agency to see if the predisposition test is required 24-48 hours prior to the haircolor service.

OBJECTIVE

To safely and effectively apply semi-permanent color to the client/guest's hair. This type of haircolor will last beyond the first cleansing treatment. **Note:** This same procedure may be utilized for a demi-permanent color application

TOOLS & MATERIALS

- Cloth and disposable towels
- Gloves
- Chemical apron
- Neck strip and cape/robe
- Color bowl and brush
- Styling brushes

- Applicator bottle
- Measuring cup
- Timer
- Color chart
- Plastic cap

- Shampoo and conditioner
- Protective cream
- Color stain remover
- Semi-permanent color
- Coloring combs

- Sectioning clips
- Cotton
- Liquid styling tools
- Thermal tools
- Client/guest record card

PROCEDURE

"The client/guest consultation is an important part of your professional service. Be sure to complete this step prior to each client/guest service you provide. Your successful retail sales and customer satisfaction rates depend upon it!"

RETAIL RE-BOOK REFERRAL

1. Cosmetologist sanitizes hands and station.
2. Set out service tools and materials.
3. Drape the client/guest in preparation for a chemical service.
4. Perform scalp and hair analysis along with preliminary strand testing.

5. Follow procedure as shown and manufacturer's instructions.
6. Follow standard cleanup procedure.
7. Document client/guest record card.

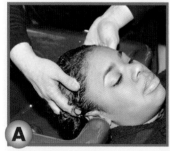

A

Lightly cleanse hair and scalp. **DO NOT** perform manipulation to avoid scalp sensitivity.

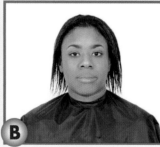

B

Towel-dry hair, absorbing any excess water.

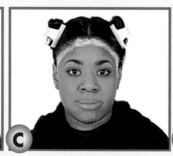

C

Divide hair into four sections and apply protective cream along hairline and ears.

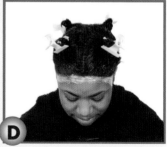

D

Outline sections and hairline with haircolor. **NOTE:** The viscosity of the color product will determine whether to use an applicator bottle or color bowl and brush.

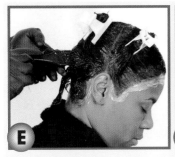

E Start in right back section, take ½ to 1 inch (1.25 cm to 2.5 cm) horizontal partings. Apply color starting at the scalp area.

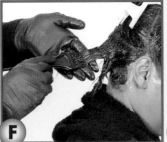

F Complete subsection by applying color on **mid-strands to hair ends** moving in a clockwise manner to the next section.

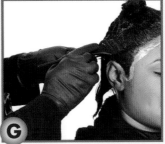

G **Repeat steps E and F** on all four sections.

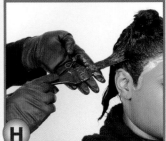

H Continue placing color from scalp, mid-strand to hair ends.

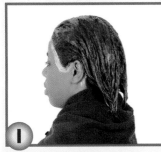

I **Complete all four sections.** Check manufacturer's instructions if color is combed through hair, if plastic cap is applied and for the processing time.

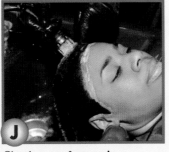

J Check manufacturer's instructions for rinsing and cleansing color from hair. Proceed with styling and finishing hair.

K Completed semi-permanent haircolor.

Permanent Haircolor Going Darker

RA

OBJECTIVE

To apply a permanent haircolor that will deposit a darker color (red) to the client/guest's existing natural level.

Before

> *Check with your local regulatory agency to see if the predisposition test is required 24-48 hours prior to the haircolor service.*

TOOLS & MATERIALS

- Cloth and disposable towels
- Gloves
- Chemical apron
- Neck strip and cape/robe
- Color bowl and brush
- Hydrometer

- Applicator bottle
- Measuring cup
- Color chart
- Plastic cap
- Timer
- Styling brushes

- Shampoo and conditioner
- Protective cream
- Color stain remover
- Permanent haircolor
- Hydrogen peroxide
- Thermal tools

- Coloring combs
- Sectioning clips
- Cotton
- Liquid styling tools
- Client/guest record card

PROCEDURE

"The client/guest consultation is an important part of your professional service. Be sure to complete this step prior to each client/guest service you provide. Your successful retail sales and customer satisfaction rates depend upon it!"

RETAIL · RE-BOOK · REFERRAL

1. Cosmetologist sanitizes hands and station.
2. Set out service tools and materials.
3. Drape client/guest in preparation for chemical service.
4. Perform scalp and hair analysis along with preliminary strand testing.
5. Follow procedure as shown and manufacturer's instructions.
6. Follow standard cleanup procedure.
7. Document client/guest record card.

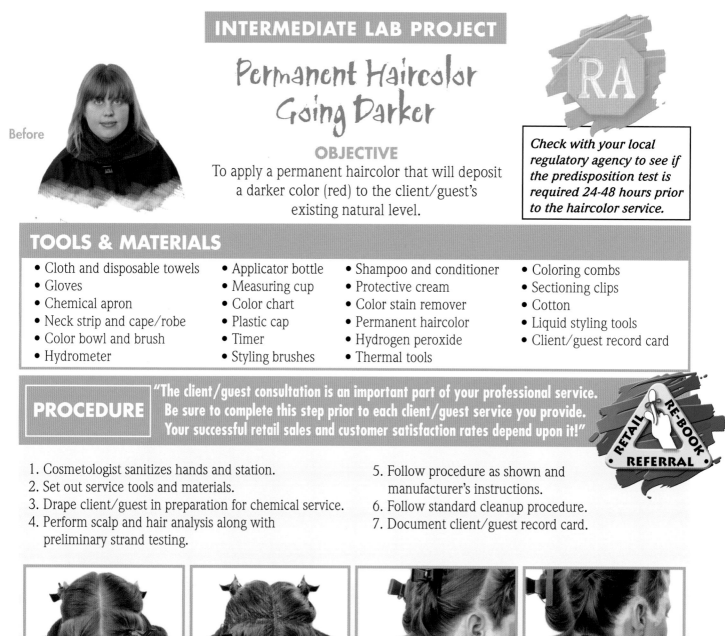

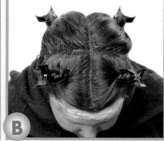 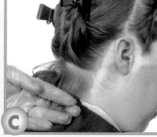 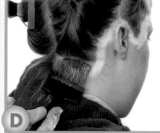

A Divide the hair into four sections. Protective cream is applied along hairline and ears.

B Outline sections and hairline with haircolor.

C Take ¼ inch (0.6 cm) **horizontal partings.**

D Begin haircolor application at the **scalp area.**

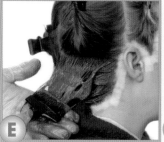 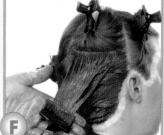 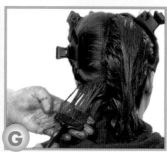 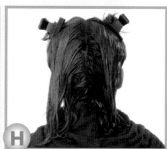

E Continue applying color over the **mid-strand to hair ends.**

F Continue taking ¼ **inch (0.6 cm) partings** and apply color from scalp to hair ends.

G **Repeat step F** to left back section.

H Completed back two sections.

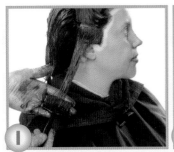

I Take ¼ inch (0.6 cm) partings at right front section and apply color from scalp to hair ends. Repeat this step to complete entire section.

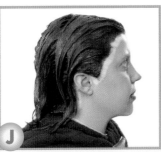

J Completed right front section.

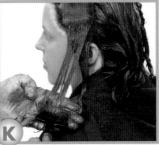

K **Repeat step I** on left front section.

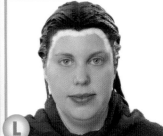

L Completed haircolor application. Process the hair following manufacturer's instructions and/or results of strand test.

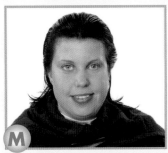

M Shampoo and condition the hair. For color staining, use cotton absorbed with color stain remover. Proceed with styling and finishing the hair.

N **Completed permanent haircolor going darker.**

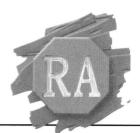

Permanent Haircolor Retouch

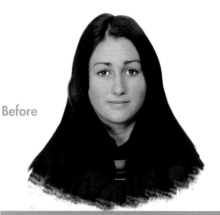

Before

OBJECTIVE
To safely and effectively apply permanent color to ONLY the client/guest's new hair growth.

Check with your local regulatory agency to see if the predisposition test is required 24-48 hours prior to the haircolor service.

TOOLS & MATERIALS

- Cloth and disposable towels
- Gloves
- Neck strip and cape/robe
- Color bowl and brush
- Chemical apron
- Hydrogen peroxide

- Applicator bottle
- Measuring cup
- Timer
- Color chart
- Thermal tools
- Styling brushes

- Plastic cap
- Shampoo and conditioner
- Protective cream
- Color stain remover
- Coloring combs
- Hydrometer

- Permanent color
- Sectioning clips
- Cotton
- Liquid styling tools
- Client/guest record card

PROCEDURE

"The client/guest consultation is an important part of your professional service. Be sure to complete this step prior to each client/guest service you provide. Your successful retail sales and customer satisfaction rates depend upon it!"

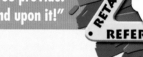

1. Cosmetologist sanitizes hands and station.
2. Set out service tools and materials.
3. Drape client/guest in preparation for chemical service.
4. Perform scalp and hair analysis along with preliminary strand testing.
5. Follow procedure as shown and manufacturer's instructions.
6. Follow standard cleanup procedure.
7. Document client/guest record card.

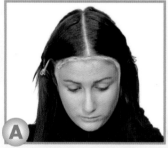

A Divide hair into four sections using a center part. Protective cream is applied along hairline and ears.

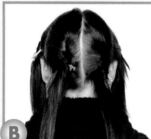

B Continue sectioning with an ear-to-ear parting.

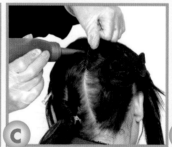

C **Outline sections and hairline** with haircolor. **NOTE:** The viscosity of the color product will determine if using an applicator bottle or color bowl and brush.

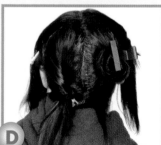

D Complete outlining the four sections with haircolor.

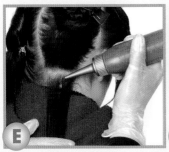

E Start in right back section, take ½ to 1 inch (1.25 cm to 2.5 cm) horizontal partings.

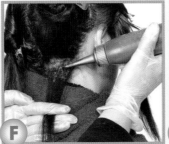

F Apply a generous amount of color **to ONLY the new growth area at scalp.**

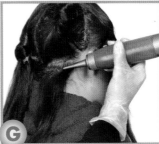

G Continue applying color to **ONLY re-growth of hair.**

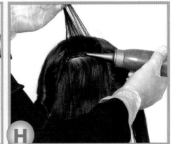

H **Repeat steps E to G** on remaining sections.

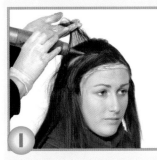

I Continue with color application to only the new growth.

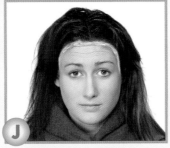

J Completed four sections. Follow manufacturer's instructions for processing time and/or results from strand test.

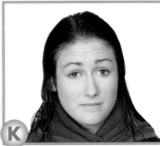

K Check manufacturer's instructions for rinsing and cleansing color from hair. Proceed with styling and finishing hair.

L Completed permanent color retouch.

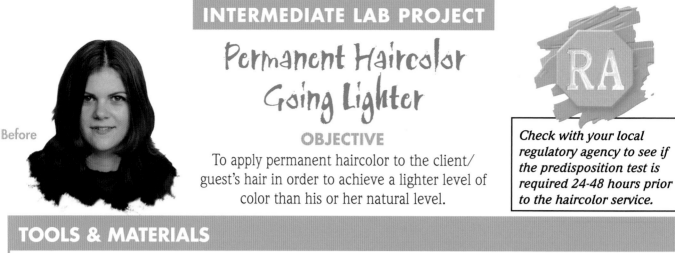

Before

Permanent Haircolor Going Lighter

OBJECTIVE

To apply permanent haircolor to the client/ guest's hair in order to achieve a lighter level of color than his or her natural level.

RA

Check with your local regulatory agency to see if the predisposition test is required 24-48 hours prior to the haircolor service.

TOOLS & MATERIALS

- Cloth and disposable towels
- Gloves
- Chemical apron
- Neck strip and cape/robe
- Color bowl and brush
- Hydrometer

- Applicator bottle
- Measuring cup
- Timer
- Color chart
- Plastic cap
- Styling brushes

- Shampoo and conditioner
- Protective cream
- Color stain remover
- Permanent haircolor
- Hydrogen peroxide
- Thermal tools

- Coloring combs
- Sectioning clips
- Cotton
- Liquid styling tools
- Client/guest record card

PROCEDURE

"The client/guest consultation is an important part of your professional service. Be sure to complete this step prior to each client/guest service you provide. Your successful retail sales and customer satisfaction rates depend upon it!"

RETAIL · RE-BOOK · REFERRAL

1. Cosmetologist sanitizes hands and station.
2. Set out service tools and materials.
3. Drape client/guest in preparation for chemical service.
4. Perform scalp and hair analysis along with preliminary strand testing.

5. Follow procedure as shown and manufacturer's instructions.
6. Follow standard cleanup procedure.
7. Document client/guest record card.

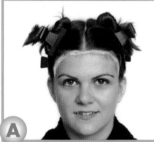

A Divide the hair into four sections. Protective cream is applied along hairline and ears.

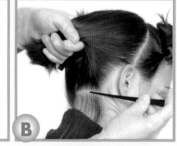

B Starting at darkest area of head, take ¼ **inch (0.6 cm) horizontal partings.**

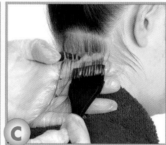

C Apply color to mid-strand, **keeping ½ to one inch (1.25 cm to 2.5 cm) away from scalp.**

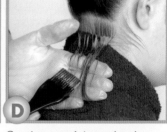

D Continue applying color down mid-strand, **keeping ½ to one inch (1.25 cm to 2.5 cm) away from hair ends.**

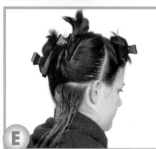

E Continue to apply color to subsections, **keeping ½ to one inch (1.25 cm to 2.5 cm) away from scalp and ends.**

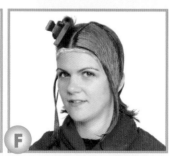

F Continue with color application working in a clockwise manner from back to front sections.

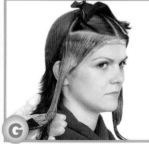

G Continue with color application, **keeping ½ to one inch (1.25 cm to 2.5 cm) away from scalp and ends.**

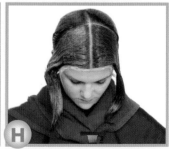

H Process the hair ⅓ **of development time** or follow manufacturer's instructions and/or results of strand test.

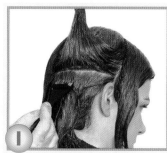

Take ¼ **inch (0.6 cm) horizontal partings,** apply color along parting at scalp area. Complete all four sections.

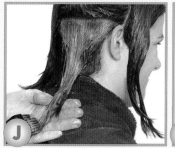

Take ¼ **inch (0.6 cm) horizontal partings,** apply color on hair ends. Complete all four sections.

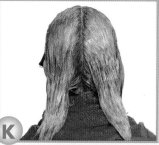

Complete color application on the two back sections.

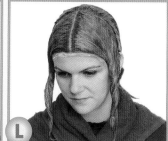

Complete color application on the two front sections.

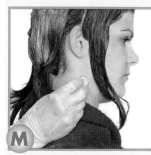

Remove color stain from neck with color stain remover.

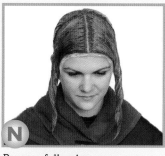

Process following manufacturer's instructions and/or results from strand test. Rinse, shampoo and condition the hair. Style and finish hair.

Completed permanent haircolor going lighter application.

Permanent Haircolor Going Lighter Retouch / Refresh

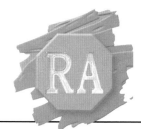

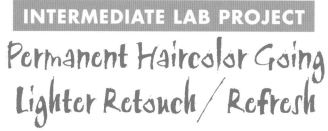

Before

OBJECTIVE

To achieve a lighter level of color by applying permanent haircolor to the client/guest's new hair growth.

> *Check with your local regulatory agency to see if the predisposition test is required 24-48 hours prior to the haircolor service.*

TOOLS & MATERIALS

- Cloth and disposable towels
- Gloves
- Chemical apron
- Neck strip and cape/robe
- Color bowl and brush
- Timer

- Applicator bottle
- Measuring cup
- Color chart
- Plastic cap
- Hydrometer
- Coloring combs

- Shampoo and conditioner
- Protective cream
- Color stain remover
- Permanent haircolor
- Hydrogen peroxide
- Styling brushes

- Thermal tools
- Sectioning clips
- Cotton
- Liquid styling tools
- Client/guest record card
- Semi- or demi-permanent haircolor

PROCEDURE

"The client/guest consultation is an important part of your professional service. Be sure to complete this step prior to each client/guest service you provide. Your successful retail sales and customer satisfaction rates depend upon it!"

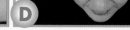

1. Cosmetologist sanitizes hands and station.
2. Set out service tools and materials.
3. Drape client/guest in preparation for chemical service.
4. Perform scalp and hair analysis along with preliminary strand testing.
5. Follow procedure as shown and manufacturer's instructions.
6. Follow standard cleanup procedure.
7. Document client/guest record card.

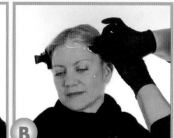

A Divide the hair into four sections.

B Apply protective cream along hairline and ears to prevent color staining.

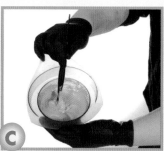

C Mix the haircolor according to the manufacturer's instructions.

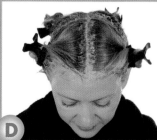

D Outline sections and hairline with color.

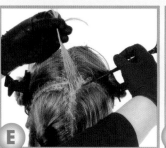

E Take ¼ **inch (0.6 cm) horizontal partings.**

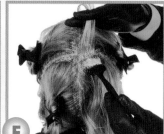

F Apply the haircolor mixture to **new growth area ONLY.**

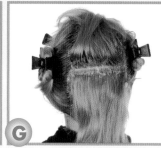

G Continue to take ¼ **inch (0.6 cm) horizontal partings** and apply color to new growth.

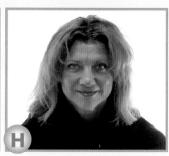

H Continue with color application working in a clockwise manner on all four sections.

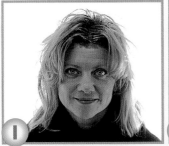

I Lift hair away from scalp for aeration to assist in color development. Process color following manufacturer's instructions and/or the results of strand test.

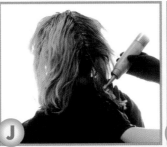

J **Optional:** To refresh remaining hair, take **¼ inch (0.6 cm) horizontal partings** and apply a semi- or demi-permanent color to mid-strand through to hair ends.

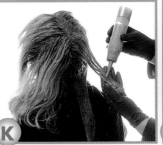

K Complete all four sections. Process and/or follow results of strand test.

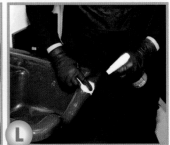

L Sanitize shampoo bowl before client/guest leans back.

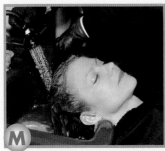

M Rinse color from hair and create a lather to assist color removal around hairline.

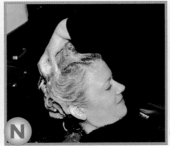

N Shampoo and condition the hair.

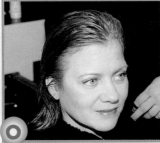

O Comb through hair and if needed, remove any color stains. Proceed with styling and finishing hair.

NOTE: When applying color to new growth, it is important **to keep 1/16 of an inch away** from previously colored hair to avoid a line of demarcation or banding. This can occur when color overlaps onto previously colored hair, resulting in a dark color band along the hair strands.

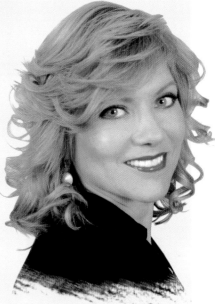

P Completed permanent haircolor going lighter retouch.

EVALUATION

GRADE   STUDENT'S NAME   ID#

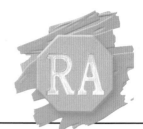

Gray Coverage Retouch

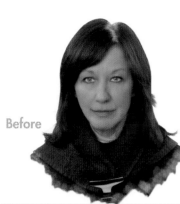

Before

OBJECTIVE

To cover gray hair by applying a permanent color to ONLY the client/ guest's new hair growth.

Check with your local regulatory agency to see if the predisposition test is required 24-48 hours prior to the haircolor service.

TOOLS & MATERIALS

- Cloth and disposable towels
- Gloves
- Chemical apron
- Neck strip and cape/robe
- Color bowl and brush
- Hydrometer

- Applicator bottle
- Measuring cup
- Timer
- Color chart
- Plastic cap
- Coloring combs

- Shampoo and conditioner
- Protective cream
- Color stain remover
- Permanent color
- Styling brushes
- Thermal tools

- Sectioning clips
- Cotton
- Liquid styling tools
- Client/guest record card

PROCEDURE

"The client/guest consultation is an important part of your professional service. Be sure to complete this step prior to each client/guest service you provide. Your successful retail sales and customer satisfaction rates depend upon it!"

RETAIL • RE-BOOK • REFERRAL

1. Cosmetologist sanitizes hands and station.
2. Set out service tools and materials.
3. Drape the client/guest in preparation for a chemical service.
4. Perform a scalp and hair analysis along with preliminary strand testing.

5. Follow procedure as shown and manufacturer's instructions.
6. Follow standard cleanup procedure.
7. Document client/guest record card.

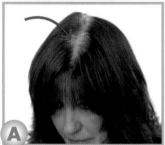

A Showing 75 percent gray hair at new growth area.

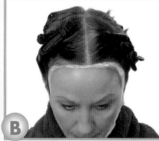

B Divide hair into four sections. Apply protective cream along hairline and ears.

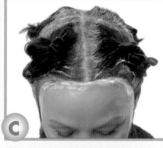

C **Outline sections and hairline** with permanent color.

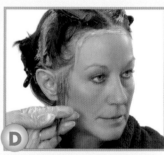

D Begin application of color at most resistant or grayest area of head. Take ¼ inch (0.6 cm) horizontal partings.

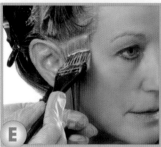

E Apply color **to ONLY the new growth area at scalp.**

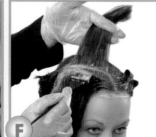

F Continue to take **¼ inch (0.6 cm) horizontal partings** and apply to new growth to complete section.

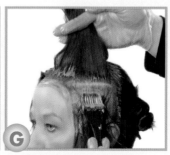

G **Repeat step F** on left front section.

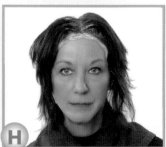

H Completed two front sections.

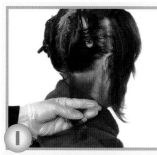

I

Take ¼ inch (0.6 cm) **horizontal partings** in right back section.

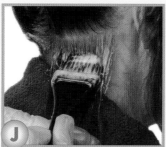

J

Apply color **to ONLY the new growth area at scalp.** Continue to apply color moving up the section.

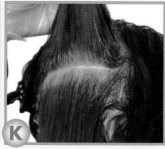

K

Showing 75 percent gray hair.

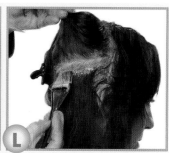

L

Repeat step J, taking ¼ inch (0.6 cm) **horizontal partings** and apply color to new growth hair.

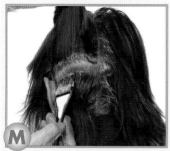

M

Repeat step L to left back section.

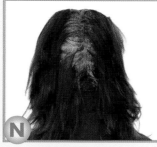

N

Completed two back sections. Follow manufacturer's instructions for processing time and/or results from strand test.

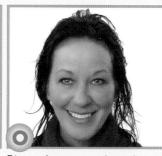

O

Rinse, shampoo and condition hair. Proceed with styling and finishing the hair.

Completed gray coverage retouch.

EVALUATION

GRADE   STUDENT'S NAME   ID#

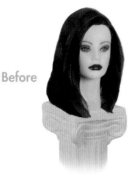

Before

COMPLEX LAB PROJECT

Double Process (Lightener with Toner)

OBJECTIVE

To effectively and safely apply hair lightener to the hair in order to diffuse the pigment to **a desired level** and then to recolorize to achieve desired haircolor result.

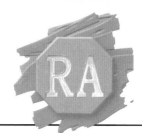

Check with your local regulatory agency to see if the predisposition test is required 24-48 hours prior to the haircolor service.

TOOLS & MATERIALS

- Cloth and disposable towels
- Gloves
- Chemical apron
- Neck strip and cape/robe
- Color bowl and brush
- Applicator bottle

- Measuring cup
- Timer
- Hydrometer
- Color chart
- Plastic cap
- Shampoo and conditioner

- Protective cream
- Color stain remover
- Hair lightener
- Hydrogen peroxide
- Haircolor product (toner)
- Coloring combs

- Styling brushes
- Sectioning clips
- Cotton
- Thermal tools
- Liquid styling tools
- Client/guest record card

PROCEDURE

"The client/guest consultation is an important part of your professional service. Be sure to complete this step prior to each client/guest service you provide. Your successful retail sales and customer satisfaction rates depend upon it!"

RETAIL • RE-BOOK • REFERRAL

1. Cosmetologist sanitizes hands and station.
2. Set out service tools and materials.
3. Drape client/guest in preparation for chemical service.
4. Perform scalp and hair analysis along with preliminary strand testing.

5. Follow procedure as shown and manufacturer's instructions.
6. Follow standard cleanup procedure.
7. Document client/guest record card.

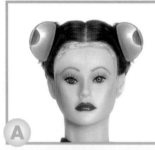

A Divide hair into four sections. Apply protective cream along hairline and ears.

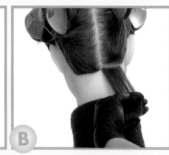

B Take ¹/₈ inch (0.3 cm) **horizontal partings.**

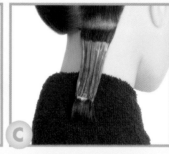

C Apply lightener on mid-strand, keep ½ to 1 inch (1.25 to 2.5 cm) away from scalp and hair ends.

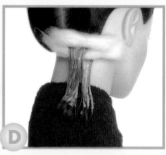

D **Optional:** Place strips of cotton between partings to prevent lightener from touching hair at scalp.

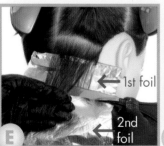

E **Optional:** Place foil between partings to prevent lightener from touching hair at scalp.

1st foil

2nd foil

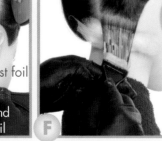

F Continue to apply lightener to subsection of hair.

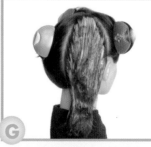

G Complete right back section with lightener application on mid-strands.

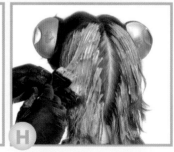

H **Repeat steps B to F** on left back section.

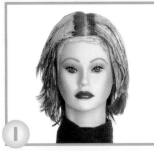

I Complete front sections with application of lightener on mid-strands.

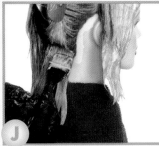

J Take ⅛ **inch (0.3 cm) partings** and apply lightener to scalp area and hair ends – use a fresh lightener mixture.

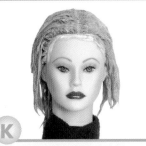

K Completed sections with lightener application. Process and strand test to determine when hair is lightened to **50 percent of the desired level.**

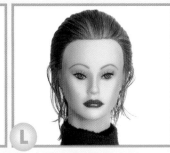

L Gently cleanse the hair to assure all lightener is removed. Towel-dry by gently blotting the hair, **no vigorous rubbing.**

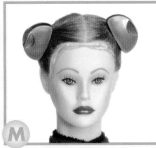

M Divide hair into four sections. Apply protective cream along hairline and ears.

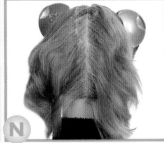

N Outline sections and hairline with color.

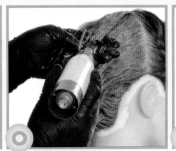

O Take ¼ **inch (0.6 cm) horizontal partings** and apply haircolor (toner) scalp to hair ends.

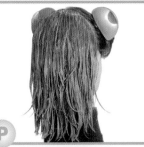

P Repeat step O to all hair sections and process following manufacturer's instructions.

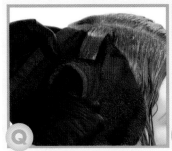

Q Strand test to determine if processing is complete.

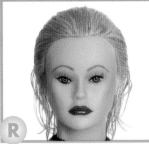

R Rinse, shampoo and condition the hair. Proceed with styling and finishing the hair.

S Completed double process (lightener with toner).

Color Correction (Tint Back)

Before

RA

OBJECTIVE

To safely and effectively return the client/guest's hair to a desired color choice.

Check with your local regulatory agency to see if the predisposition test is required 24-48 hours prior to the haircolor service.

TOOLS & MATERIALS

- Cloth and disposable towels
- Gloves
- Chemical apron
- Neck strip and cape/robe
- Color bowl and brush
- Applicator bottle

- Measuring cup
- Timer
- Hydrometer
- Color chart
- Plastic cap
- Shampoo and conditioner

- Protective cream
- Color stain remover
- Hydrogen peroxide
- Haircolor product
- Sectioning clips
- Cotton

- Coloring combs
- Styling brushes
- Liquid styling tools
- Thermal tools
- Client/guest record card

PROCEDURE

"The client/guest consultation is an important part of your professional service. Be sure to complete this step prior to each client/guest service you provide. Your successful retail sales and customer satisfaction rates depend upon it!"

RETAIL · RE-BOOK · REFERRAL

1. Cosmetologist sanitizes hands and station.
2. Set out service tools and materials.
3. Drape client/guest in preparation for chemical service.
4. Perform scalp and hair analysis along with preliminary strand testing.

5. Follow procedure as shown and manufacturer's instructions.
6. Follow standard cleanup procedure.
7. Document client/guest record card.

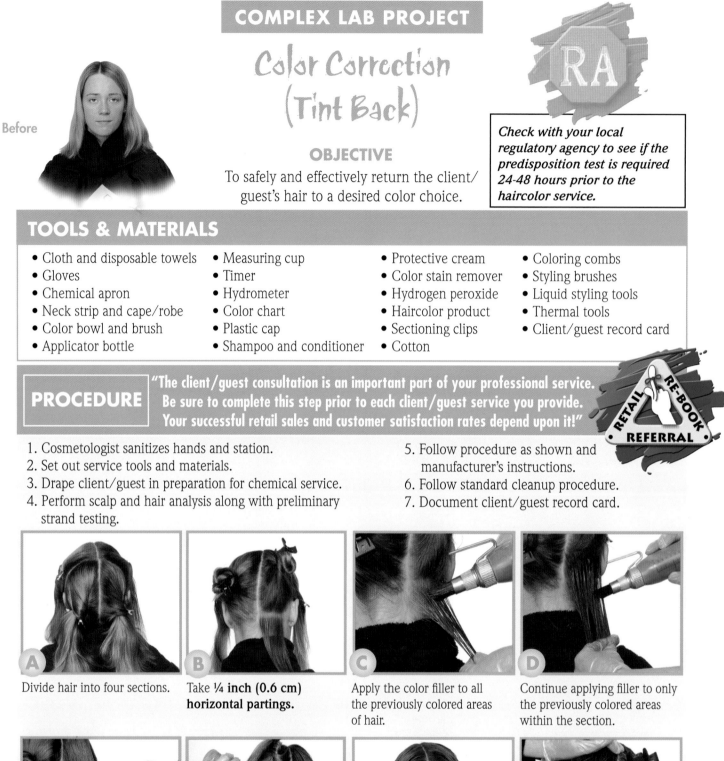

A Divide hair into four sections.

B Take ¼ inch (0.6 cm) **horizontal partings.**

C Apply the color filler to all the previously colored areas of hair.

D Continue applying filler to only the previously colored areas within the section.

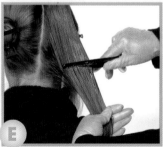

E **Optional:** Comb through hair to evenly distribute color – follow manufacturer's instructions.

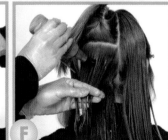

F **Repeat steps B to E** on all four sections.

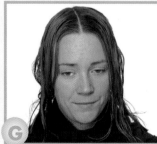

G Complete all four sections – strand test to determine haircolor absorption and processing. **DO NOT remove filler from hair.**

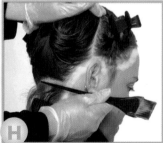

H Apply protective cream along hairline and ears. Re-divide the hair into four sections, take ¼ inch (0.6 cm) **horizontal partings.**

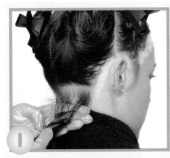

I Apply color on mid-strand of parting, keep ½ to 1 inch (1.25 cm to 2.5 cm) away from the scalp.

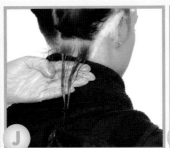

J Keep color ½ to 1 inch (1.25 cm to 2.5 cm) away from the hair ends.

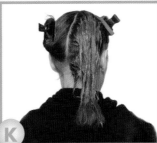

K Continue to apply color to remaining section.

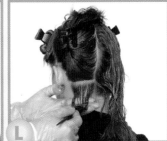

L Complete color application on all four sections.

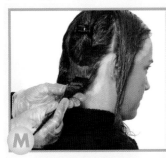

M Return to right back section and **apply color to scalp and hair ends.**

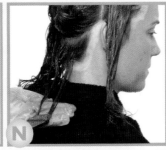

N Apply color to hair ends. Complete all four sections following **steps M and N.**

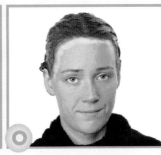

O Follow manufacturer's instructions for processing and/or the results of the strand test.

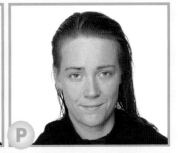

P Rinse, shampoo and condition hair – proceed with styling and finishing hair.

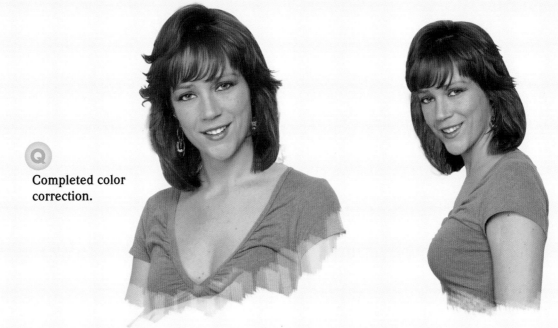

Q Completed color correction.

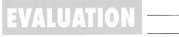

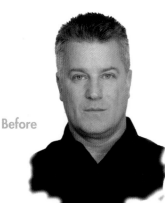

Before

Five-Minute Haircoloring

OBJECTIVE

To apply an alternative type of haircolor that **processes in five minutes** and provides color, but not over-all coverage. This category of haircolor falls under either semi-permanent or demi-permanent color depending on manufacturer.

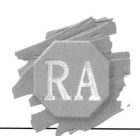

Check with your local regulatory agency to see if the predisposition test is required 24-48 hours prior to the haircolor service.

TOOLS & MATERIALS

- Cloth and disposable towels
- Gloves
- Chemical apron
- Neck strip and cape/robe
- Color bowl and brush
- Applicator bottle
- Hydrometer
- Measuring cup
- Timer
- Color chart
- Plastic cap
- Coloring combs
- Shampoo and conditioner
- Protective cream
- Color stain remover
- Haircolor product
- Hydrogen peroxide
- Styling brushes
- Thermal tools
- Sectioning clips
- Cotton
- Liquid styling tools
- Client/guest record card

PROCEDURE

"The client/guest consultation is an important part of your professional service. Be sure to complete this step prior to each client/guest service you provide. Your successful retail sales and customer satisfaction rates depend upon it!"

RETAIL RE-BOOK REFERRAL

1. Cosmetologist sanitizes hands and station.
2. Set out service tools and materials.
3. Drape client/guest in preparation for chemical service.
4. Perform scalp and hair analysis along with preliminary strand testing.
5. Follow procedure as shown and manufacturer's instructions.
6. Follow standard cleanup procedure.
7. Document client/guest record card.

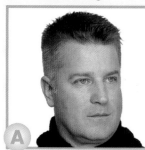

A Client/guest's hair appearing **50 percent gray** on sides of head.

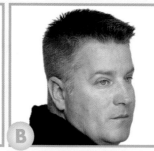

B Side view showing **over 50 percent gray** at **sideburn area.**

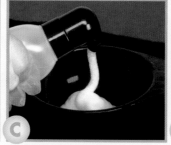

C Squeeze or place color product into coloring bowl or applicator bottle. **NOTE:** Notice consistency of product.

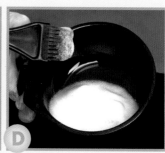

D Immerse color brush into product – sudsy and foam consistency.

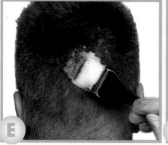

E Apply haircolor to back of head or most resistant area. No sectioning required due to short-length hair.

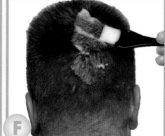

F Continue with color application over occipital of head.

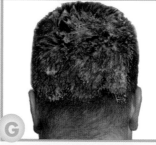

G Completed color application to occipital area of head.

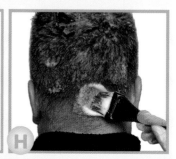

H Apply haircolor to nape area (gray) of head.

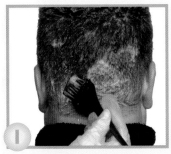

Continue with application of haircolor to hair at nape.

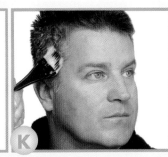

Completed color application to back of head.

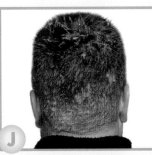

Apply haircolor to sides of head and top of head.

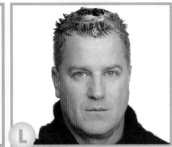

Completed color application to top of head.

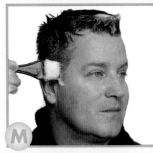

Apply haircolor to **grayest area – sideburn hair.**

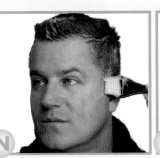

Repeat color application on opposite side of head.

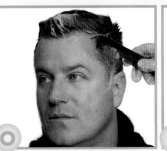

Comb through hair using a large-tooth comb, starting on top of head moving down over sides of head.

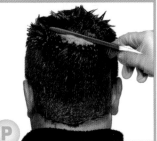

Continue to comb over entire head to ensure even color absorption.

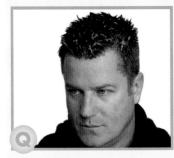

Completed haircolor application over entire head.

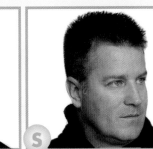

Side view of color application. **Process for five minutes.**

Rinse, shampoo and condition hair. Style and finish hair.

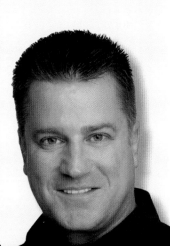

T **Completed five-minute haircolor.**

NOTE: This type of color is great for men that want an undetected haircolor change with a natural appearance.

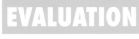

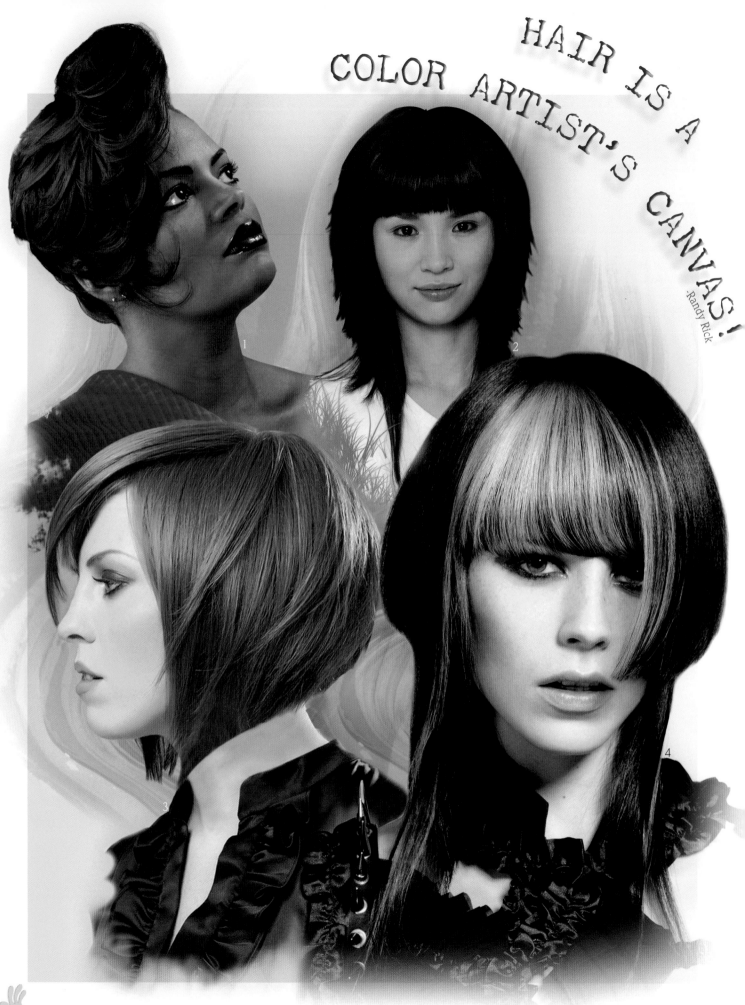

HAIR IS A
COLOR ARTIST'S CANVAS!
-Randy Rick

foils

dimensional

highlights

lowlights

patterns

weaving

zones

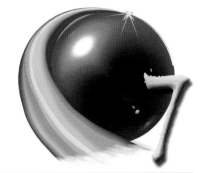

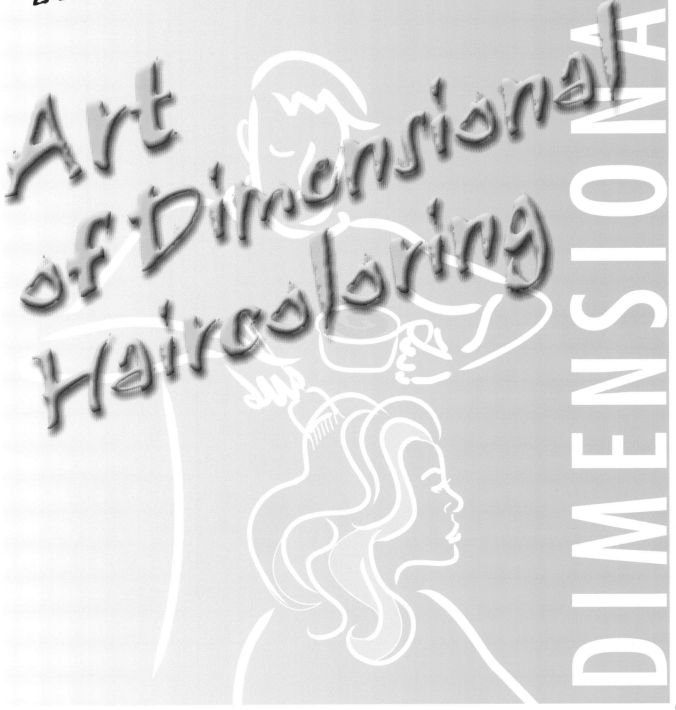

Art
of Dimensional
Haircoloring

DIMENSIONAL

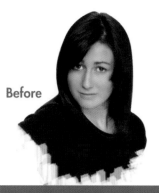
Before

Free Hand Painting

OBJECTIVE

To create a subtle dimensional effect by free-form painting lightener and/or haircolor on selected hair strands of the hairdesign.

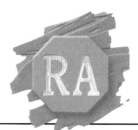

Check with your local regulatory agency to see if the predisposition test is required 24-48 hours prior to the haircolor service.

TOOLS & MATERIALS

- Cloth and disposable towels
- Gloves
- Chemical apron
- Neck strip and cape/robe
- Color bowl and brush
- Paddle brush
- Measuring cup
- Timer
- Hydrometer
- Color chart
- Shampoo and conditioner
- Color stain remover
- Hair and color combs
- Hair lightener
- Hydrogen peroxide
- Haircolor product
- Protective cream
- Coloring combs
- Thermal tools
- Sectioning clips
- Cotton
- Liquid styling tools
- Client/guest record card

PROCEDURE

"The client/guest consultation is an important part of your professional service. Be sure to complete this step prior to each client/guest service you provide. Your successful retail sales and customer satisfaction rates depend upon it!"

RETAIL RE-BOOK REFERRAL

1. Cosmetologist sanitizes hands and station.
2. Set out service tools and materials.
3. Drape client/guest in preparation for chemical service.
4. Perform scalp/hair analysis along with preliminary strand testing.
5. Follow procedure as shown and manufacturer's instructions.
6. Follow standard cleanup procedure.
7. Document client/guest record card.

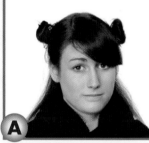

A Section hair following client/guest's desired hairdesign.

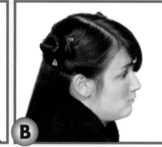

B Side view of the sectioning pattern.

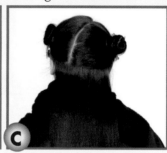

C Part a **2 to 3 inch (5 to 7.6 cm) subsection** of hair and comb smooth. Mix lightener following manufacturer's instructions.

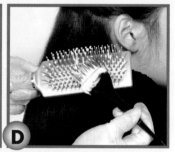

D **Place lightener over the ends of the bristles** on a paddle brush.

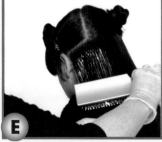

E **Place bristles of brush on hair with slight penetration** and move down toward hair ends. The amount of lightener applied depends on end result.

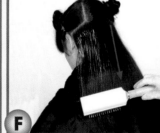

F **Glide brush downward through strands to hair ends.** Remove brush and re-position on next area of subsection.

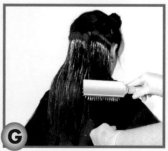

G Repeat **steps E and F** to the remaining subsection. More lightener is applied on the bristles as needed.

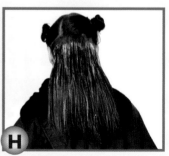

H Complete subsection using lightener.

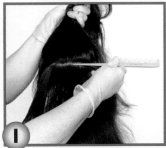

I Divide another **2 to 3 inch (5 to 7.6 cm) horizontal subsection** of hair and comb smooth. **In separate bowls, mix a warm and a cool red color.**

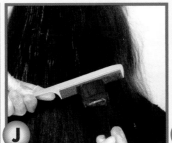

J Apply the **cool red color on teeth of tail comb.**

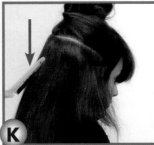

K **Place teeth of the comb in a vertical position and glide** down the length of hair. Repeat throughout subsection.

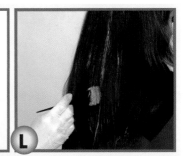

L Apply **warm red color using the tint brush**; place color between two cool red colors gliding down length of hair. Repeat throughout subsection.

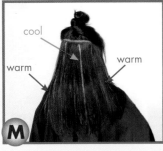

M Alternate between the warm and cool red throughout subsection. Add more product to teeth of comb as needed.

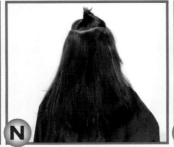

N Divide another **2 to 3 inch (5 to 7.6 cm) horizontal subsection** of hair and comb smooth.

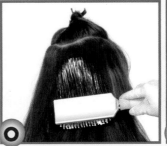

O Apply lightener using the paddle brush – **repeat steps D thru H.**

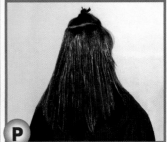

P Complete the subsection with lightener application.

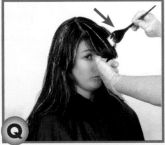

Q Comb down last subsection of hair (including fringe area) and apply lightener using tint brush.

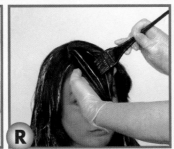

R Continue by placing the warm and cool red colors alternating between the two. Add more product to teeth as needed.

S Completed application of lightener with both red colors. Process following manufacturer's directions, strand test, rinse, shampoo and condition hair. Proceed with styling and finishing.

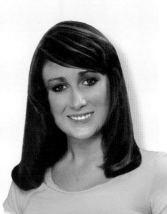

T **Completed free hand painting.**

NOTE: This technique of color application is sometimes referred to as **Baliage** (ba-lay-age), which is a French term meaning, "strands of color."

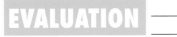

Highlighting with Cap and Hook

Before

OBJECTIVE

To deliver a fast method of selecting and preparing short length hair strands that will be colored and/ or lightened to create a contrasting finish.

RA

Check with your local regulatory agency to see if the predisposition test is required 24-48 hours prior to the haircolor service.

TOOLS & MATERIALS

- Cloth and disposable towels
- Gloves
- Chemical apron
- Neck strip and cape/robe
- Color bowl and brush
- Applicator bottle

- Measuring cup
- Timer
- Hydrometer
- Color chart
- Plastic cap
- Shampoo and conditioner

- Protective cream
- Color stain remover
- Hair lightener
- Hydrogen peroxide
- Haircolor product (high-lift)
- Coloring combs

- Sectioning clips
- Cotton
- Liquid styling tools
- Thermal tools
- Haircoloring cap/hook
- Client/guest record card

PROCEDURE

"The client/guest consultation is an important part of your professional service. Be sure to complete this step prior to each client/guest service you provide. Your successful retail sales and customer satisfaction rates depend upon it!"

RETAIL RE-BOOK REFERRAL

1. Cosmetologist sanitizes hands and station.
2. Set out service tools and materials.
3. Drape client/guest in preparation for chemical service.
4. Perform scalp/hair analysis along with preliminary strand testing.
5. Follow procedure as shown and manufacturer's instructions.
6. Follow standard cleanup procedure.
7. Document client/guest record card.

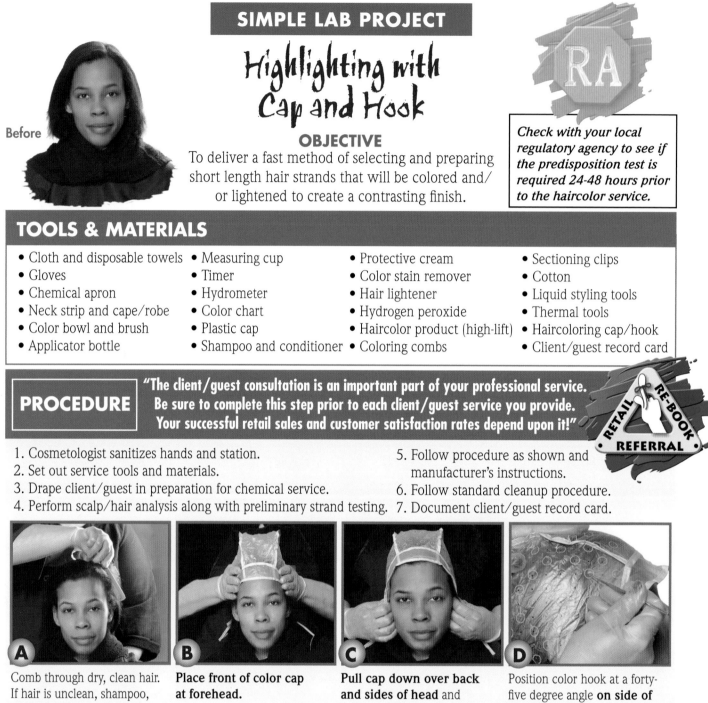

A Comb through dry, clean hair. If hair is unclean, shampoo, condition and dry hair before placement of color cap.

B **Place front of color cap at forehead.**

C **Pull cap down over back and sides of head** and secure. *(Refer to Chapter 2 for other alternatives in color cap positioning.)*

D Position color hook at a forty-five degree angle **on side of head at the hairline.**

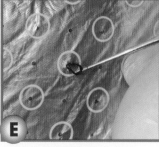

E **Use clasp of color hook to gently pierce plastic and grasp some hair.**

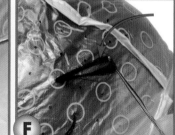

F **Gently pull hair through hole.**

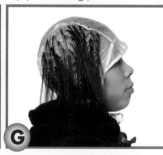

G Continue pulling hair through holes on sides of head. Amount of hair pulled depends on desired end result.

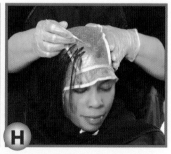

H Continue on top and center panel of color cap – stay consistent with amount of hair pulled from each hole.

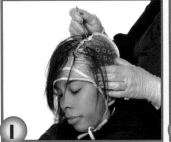

I Complete pulling hair from holes on opposite side of head.

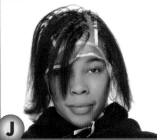

J Comb hair to remove tangles and keep smooth. Mix lightener or a high-lift color following manufacturer's directions.

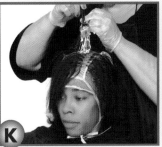

K Start applying product to the hair at **crown area** (this is the recommended area to begin application).

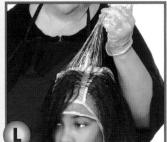

L Apply lightener on both sides of hair strands to ensure even coverage and absorption.

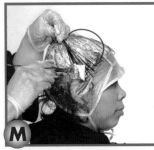

M Continue to **apply product moving in a clockwise manner** around the head.

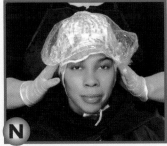

N Complete application of lightener on the head. Cover hair with plastic bag and secure – check manufacturer's directions.

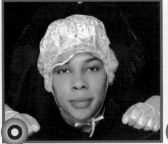

O Process following manufacturer's directions and/or preliminary strand testing results.

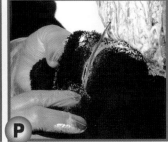

P Strand test to check degree of lightness. Once desired color is reached, do not remove cap, rinse hair first, and then remove color cap, shampoo, condition and dry hair.

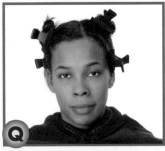

Q **Optional:** If desiring additional haircolor to cover all hair, re-section dry hair.

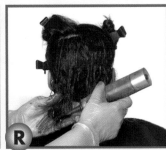

R Apply color from scalp to hair ends taking ¼ **inch (0.6 cm) partings**. Process following manufacturer's directions and/or strand test results.

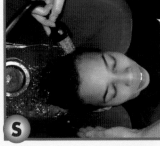

S Rinse, shampoo and condition hair. Proceed with styling and finishing.

NOTE: If haircolor is applied to ONLY hair pulled through cap, rinse and shampoo the hair, towel-dry – **DO NOT remove color cap;** apply color and process.

T Completed highlight with cap and hook.

EVALUATION

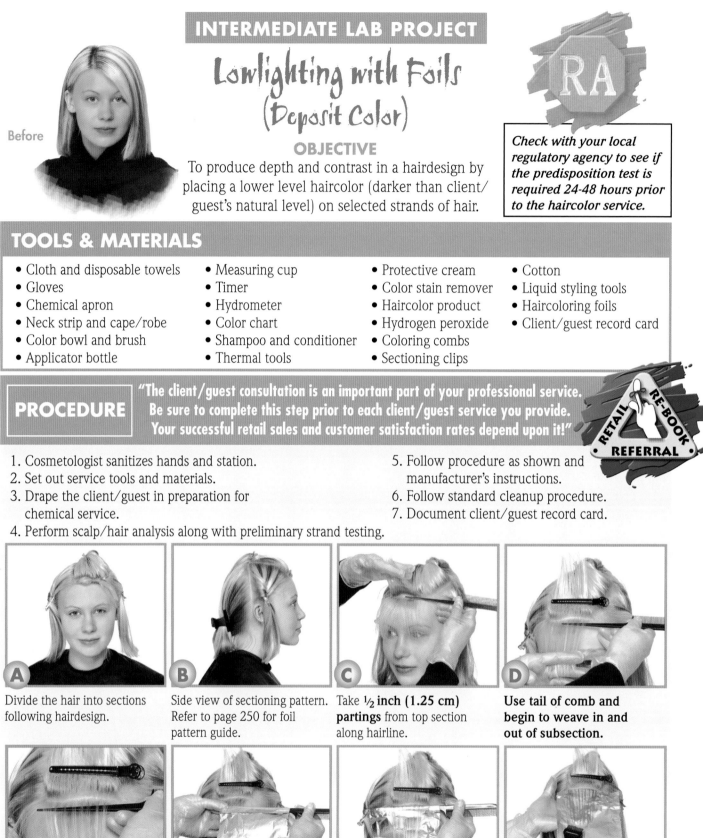

Lowlighting with Foils
(Deposit Color)

Before

RA

OBJECTIVE
To produce depth and contrast in a hairdesign by placing a lower level haircolor (darker than client/guest's natural level) on selected strands of hair.

Check with your local regulatory agency to see if the predisposition test is required 24-48 hours prior to the haircolor service.

TOOLS & MATERIALS

- Cloth and disposable towels
- Gloves
- Chemical apron
- Neck strip and cape/robe
- Color bowl and brush
- Applicator bottle

- Measuring cup
- Timer
- Hydrometer
- Color chart
- Shampoo and conditioner
- Thermal tools

- Protective cream
- Color stain remover
- Haircolor product
- Hydrogen peroxide
- Coloring combs
- Sectioning clips

- Cotton
- Liquid styling tools
- Haircoloring foils
- Client/guest record card

PROCEDURE

"The client/guest consultation is an important part of your professional service. Be sure to complete this step prior to each client/guest service you provide. Your successful retail sales and customer satisfaction rates depend upon it!"

RETAIL • RE-BOOK • REFERRAL

1. Cosmetologist sanitizes hands and station.
2. Set out service tools and materials.
3. Drape the client/guest in preparation for chemical service.
4. Perform scalp/hair analysis along with preliminary strand testing.
5. Follow procedure as shown and manufacturer's instructions.
6. Follow standard cleanup procedure.
7. Document client/guest record card.

A Divide the hair into sections following hairdesign.

B Side view of sectioning pattern. Refer to page 250 for foil pattern guide.

C Take ½ inch (1.25 cm) **partings** from top section along hairline.

D Use tail of comb and begin to weave in and out of subsection.

E Amount of hair weaved out of subsection (for this design) is ¼ inch (0.6 cm) deep – determined by desired end result.

F Insert tail of comb inside fold at end of foil.

G Place foil underneath subsection, withdraw comb and hold foil against scalp using fingers of the opposite hand.

H Apply a medium warm red color to all the hair on the foil.

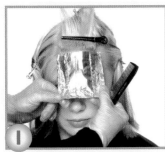

I Secure hair by folding foil in half and turning sides into center.

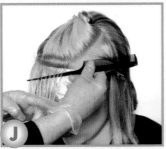

J Part a ½ inch (1.25 cm) **subsection** of hair between each foil packet and weave a ¼ inch (0.6 cm) deep into hair.

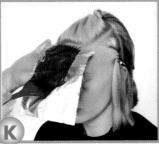

K Place foil underneath subsection of hair, **apply a medium cool red color** and secure foil.

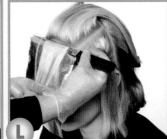

L Part a ½ inch (1.25 cm) **subsection** and slice ¼ inch (0.6 cm) and place hair on foil.

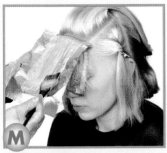

M **Apply a light warm red color** to hair on foil. Continue red color pattern by repeating **steps H, K and M** to complete the top section.

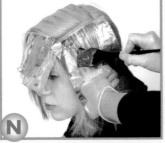

N **Follow color pattern of medium warm red (weave), cool red (weave) and light warm red (slice).**

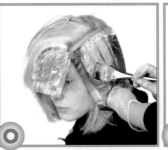

O Continue to repeat the red color pattern to both side sections.

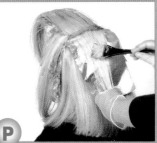

P Repeat **steps N and O** on back sections.

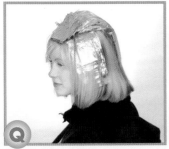

Q Completed hair sections with color packets. Process following manufacturer's directions and/or results of strand test.

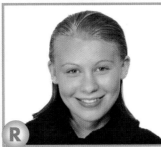

R Remove foils, rinse, shampoo and condition hair. Proceed with styling and finishing hair.

S Completed lowlighting with foils.

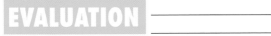

Highlighting with Foils (Partial)

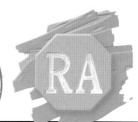

RA

Before

OBJECTIVE

To produce contrast on a partial area of the hairdesign by placing a lightener or high level haircolor (lighter than client/guest's natural level or tone) on selected strands of hair.

Check with your local regulatory agency to see if the predisposition test is required 24-48 hours prior to the haircolor service.

TOOLS & MATERIALS

- Cloth and disposable towels
- Gloves
- Chemical apron
- Neck strip and cape/robe
- Color bowl and brush
- Applicator bottle

- Measuring cup
- Timer
- Hydrometer
- Color chart
- Shampoo and conditioner
- Protective cream

- Color stain remover
- Hair lightener
- Hydrogen peroxide
- Haircolor product
- Coloring combs
- Thermal tools

- Sectioning clips
- Cotton
- Liquid styling tools
- Haircoloring foils
- Client/guest record card

PROCEDURE

"The client/guest consultation is an important part of your professional service. Be sure to complete this step prior to each client/guest service you provide. Your successful retail sales and customer satisfaction rates depend upon it!"

RETAIL · RE-BOOK · REFERRAL

1. Cosmetologist sanitizes hands and station.
2. Set out service tools and materials.
3. Drape the client/guest in preparation for a chemical service.
4. Perform scalp/hair analysis along with preliminary strand testing.
5. Follow procedure as shown and manufacturer's instructions.
6. Follow standard cleanup procedure.
7. Document client/guest record card

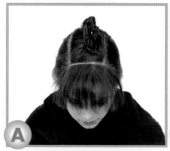

A Divide top section (top view) **ONLY.**

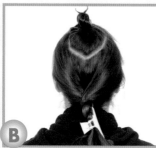

B Top section (back view). Refer to page 251 for foil pattern guide.

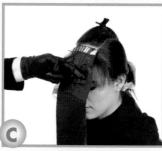

C Take a ½ inch (1.25 cm) parting, weave 1/16 to 1/8 inch (0.15 cm to 0.3 cm) deep and place hair on foil.

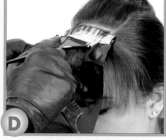

D Apply lightener from scalp to hair ends, secure foil. Repeat steps C and D to entire section.

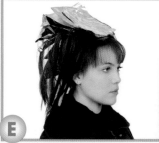

E Complete top section with foils. Process until desired level of lightness is achieved and perform a strand test.

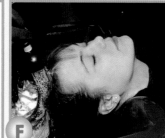

F Remove foils and rinse hair.

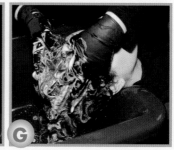

G Lightly shampoo the hair – no scalp manipulations.

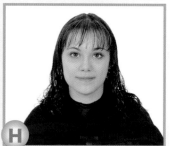

H Towel-dry and comb through hair.

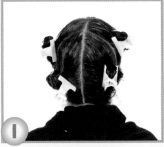

I Divide hair into four sections.

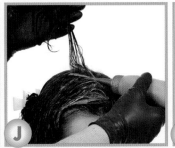

J Take ½ **inch (1.25 cm) partings** and **apply toner ONLY on highlighted area of head** from scalp to hair ends.

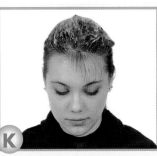

K Complete toner application. Process following manufacturer's directions and/or results of strand test.

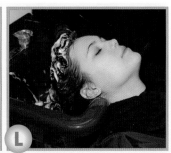

L Rinse, shampoo and condition hair.

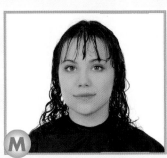

M Comb through and proceed with styling and finishing.

N Completed partial highlights with foils.

Highlighting with Foils (Full)

RA

OBJECTIVE

To produce contrast in an over-all hairdesign by placing a lightener or high level haircolor (lighter than client/guest's natural level or tone) on selected strands of hair using foil.

Check with your local regulatory agency to see if the predisposition test is required 24-48 hours prior to the haircolor service.

Before

TOOLS & MATERIALS

- Cloth and disposable towels
- Gloves
- Chemical apron
- Neck and strip and cape/robe
- Color bowl and brush
- Applicator bottle

- Measuring cup
- Timer
- Color chart
- Hydrometer
- Shampoo and conditioner
- Protective cream

- Color stain remover
- Hair lightener
- Hydrogen peroxide
- Haircolor product
- Coloring combs
- Thermal tools

- Sectioning clips
- Cotton
- Liquid styling tools
- Haircoloring foils
- Client/guest record card

PROCEDURE

"The client/guest consultation is an important part of your professional service. Be sure to complete this step prior to each client/guest service you provide. Your successful retail sales and customer satisfaction rates depend upon it!"

RETAIL • RE-BOOK • REFERRAL

1. Cosmetologist sanitizes hands and station.
2. Set out service tools and materials.
3. Drape client/guest in preparation for chemical service.
4. Perform scalp/hair analysis along with preliminary strand testing.
5. Follow procedure as shown and manufacturer's instructions.
6. Follow standard cleanup procedure.
7. Document client/guest record card.

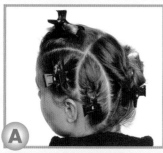

A Shows hair divided into a standard nine sections – may use any sectioning pattern desired. Refer to page 252 for foil pattern guide.

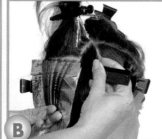

B Take ½ **inch (1.25 cm) parting** with a ½ **inch deep weave** from center back section. Amount of hair used depends on texture and desired end result.

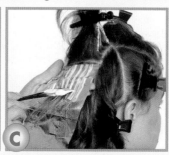

C Apply lightener on the hair close to the scalp. **DO NOT place lightener directly on the scalp** to avoid discoloration due to body heat creating product leakage.

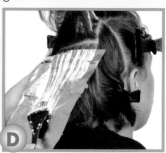

D Continue applying lightener to remaining hair.

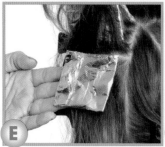

E Secure hair by folding foil in half and turning sides into center.

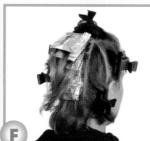

F Complete back center section. Amount of hair taken between each packet is ½ **inch (1.25 cm).**

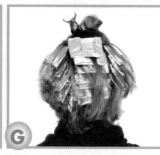

G Complete the two side back panels following **steps B to F**.

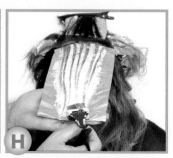

H Continue with ½ **inch (1.25 cm) partings** and a ½ **inch deep weave** on top center section and applying lightener.

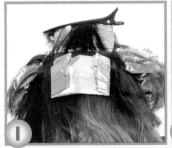

I — Secure hair by folding foil in half and turning sides into center.

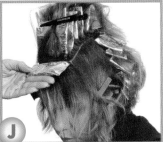

J — Continue placing lightener on selected subsections of hair working down toward hairline.

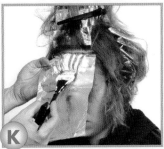

K — Apply lightener from scalp area to hair ends and complete the center top section.

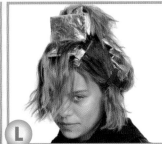

L — Completed top center section.

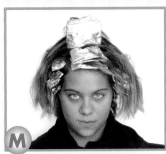

M — Complete the remaining side front sections following **steps H to K.**

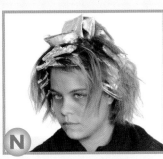

N — Completed top and side sections. Process following manufacturer's directions and/or results of strand test. Remove foils and rinse, shampoo, condition hair. Style and finish hair.

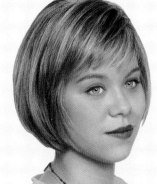

O — Completed **full highlighting with foils.**

Highlighting using Crisscross Pattern

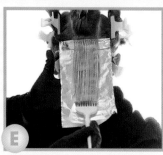

Before

OBJECTIVE
To create contrast in a hairdesign by placing a lightener or high level haircolor on selected strands of hair using a crisscross technique.

RA

Check with your local regulatory agency to see if the predisposition test is required 24-48 hours prior to the haircolor service.

TOOLS & MATERIALS

- Cloth and disposable towels
- Gloves
- Chemical apron
- Neck strip and cape/robe
- Color bowl and brush
- Applicator bottle

- Measuring cup
- Timer
- Hydrometer
- Color chart
- Shampoo and conditioner
- Protective cream

- Color stain remover
- Hair lightener
- Hydrogen peroxide
- Haircolor product
- Coloring combs
- Thermal tools

- Sectioning clips
- Cotton
- Liquid styling tools
- Haircoloring foils
- Client/guest record card

PROCEDURE

"The client/guest consultation is an important part of your professional service. Be sure to complete this step prior to each client/guest service you provide. Your successful retail sales and customer satisfaction rates depend upon it!"

RETAIL RE-BOOK REFERRAL

1. Cosmetologist sanitizes hands and station.
2. Set out service tools and materials.
3. Drape client/guest in preparation for chemical service.
4. Perform a scalp and hair analysis along with preliminary strand testing.
5. Follow procedure as shown and manufacturer's instructions.
6. Follow standard cleanup procedure.
7. Document client/guest record card.

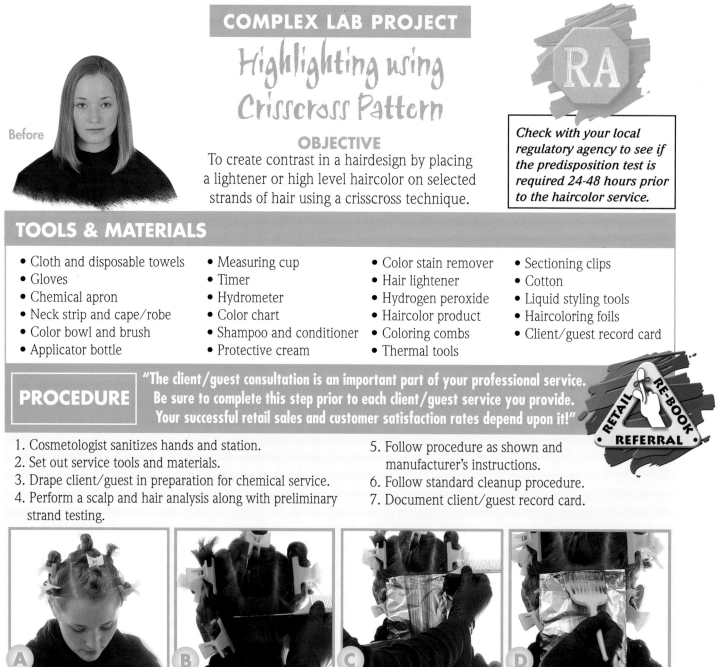

A Divide the hair into nine sections to complete a crisscross pattern. Refer to page 253 for foil pattern guide.

B Slice ⅛ to ¼ inch (0.3 to 0.6 cm) horizontal parting of hair.

C Place foil under subsection of hair.

D Apply lightener on hair close to scalp. **DO NOT place lightener directly on scalp** to avoid product leakage due to body heat.

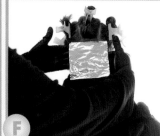

E Continue lightener application to remaining hair.

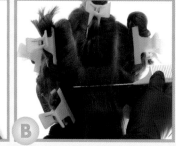

F Secure foil by folding in half. **Optional:** Depending on length of foil, repeat folding foil in half.

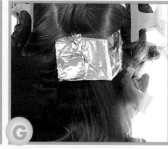

G Fold sides into center of foil.

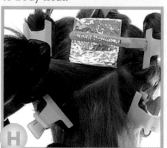

H Take a ½ inch to one inch (1.25 to 2.5 cm) diagonal parting. This hair receives no lightener.

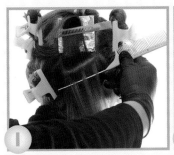

Weave hair ½ inch to one inch (1.25 cm) deep. Amount of hair selected for weave is determined by desired end result.

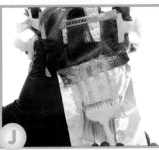

Apply lightener from scalp to hair ends and secure foil. Divide ½ inch (1.25 cm) **diagonal parting between each foil packet; do not apply product to this subsection of hair.**

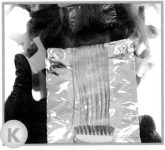

Divide another **diagonal sliced parting of hair,** place under foil, apply lightener and secure foil.

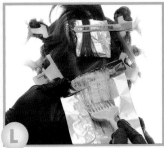

Continue foil pattern; alternating between diagonal weave and sliced partings to remaining section.

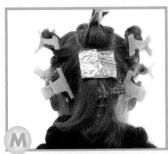

Complete section with crisscross foil pattern. Repeat **steps B to L** on remaining sections.

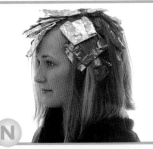

All sections completed. Process following manufacturer's directions and/or results of strand test. Remove foils, rinse, shampoo and condition.

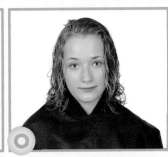

Towel-dry and comb through hair. Style and finish the hair.

P **Completed highlights with crisscross pattern.**

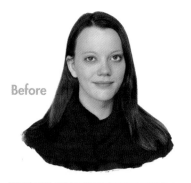

Before

Tone-on-Tone Coloring

OBJECTIVE

To create a subtle tone-on-tone hairdesign by adding soft golden blonde and warm auburn colors to natural light/medium brown hair.

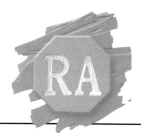

RA

Check with your local regulatory agency to see if the predisposition test is required 24-48 hours prior to the haircolor service.

TOOLS & MATERIALS

- Cloth and disposable towels
- Gloves
- Chemical apron
- Neck strip and cape/robe
- Color bowl and brush
- Applicator bottle

- Measuring cup
- Timer
- Hydrometer
- Color chart
- Shampoo and conditioner
- Protective cream

- Color stain remover
- Hair lightener
- Hydrogen peroxide
- Haircolor product
- Coloring combs
- Haircoloring foils

- Thermal tools
- Sectioning clips
- Cotton
- Liquid styling tools
- Client/guest record card

PROCEDURE

"The client/guest consultation is an important part of your professional service. Be sure to complete this step prior to each client/guest service you provide. Your successful retail sales and customer satisfaction rates depend upon it!"

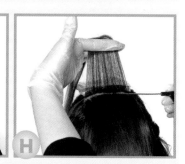

RETAIL · RE-BOOK · REFERRAL

1. Cosmetologist sanitizes hands and station.
2. Set out service tools and materials.
3. Drape client/guest in preparation for chemical service.
4. Perform a scalp and hair analysis along with preliminary strand testing.
5. Follow procedure as shown and manufacturer's instructions.
6. Follow standard cleanup procedure.
7. Document client/guest record card.

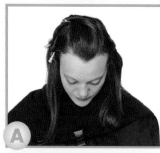

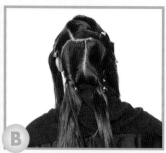

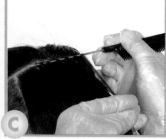

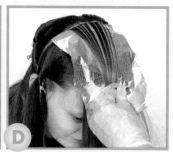

A Divide the hair into sections following client/guest's hairdesign.

B Back view of sectioning pattern. Refer to page 254 for foil pattern guide.

C Amount of hair selected for **weave is ¼ to ½ inch (0.6 to 1.25 cm) deep.**

D Place weaved hair on top of foil.

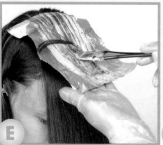

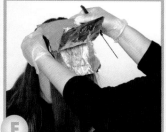

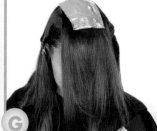

E **Apply lightener** on full length of weaved hair.

F Secure hair by placing an additional piece of foil on top of hair.

G Fold foil in half with sides turned into center.

H Part a ½ inch (1.25 cm) subsection of hair; do not apply product.

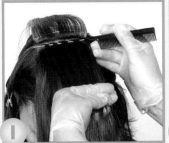

I Continue to **weave ¼ to ½ inch (0.6 to 1.25 cm) amount of hair.**

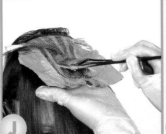

J Apply **medium auburn color** from scalp to hair ends. Fold to secure foil.

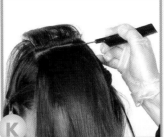

K Part another ½ inch (1.25 cm) of hair; do not apply product.

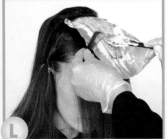

L **Slice a ¼ inch (0.6 cm) parting,** place foil and apply lightener. Fold to secure foil.

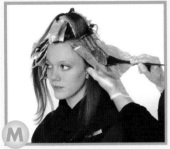

M **Continue foil pattern to top and side sections : first foil – weave hair and apply lightener, second foil – weave hair and apply color, third foil – slice hair and apply lightener; repeat color pattern.**

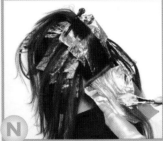

N Complete back section repeating the same color pattern.

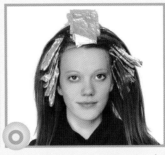

O Completed full head color/ lightener application.

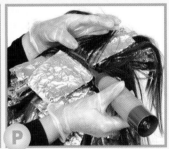

P **Apply a dark warm red color to remaining hair not in the foil –** start at scalp area.

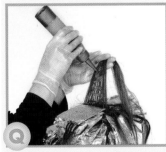

Q Continue applying color to mid-strand and hair ends.

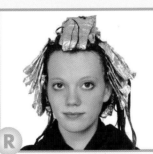

R Complete dark warm red color to remaining hair. Process and perform strand test. Remove foils, rinse, shampoo and condition hair. Proceed with styling and finishing hair.

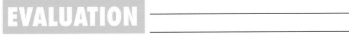

S **Completed tone-on-tone coloring.**

Ribbons of Color

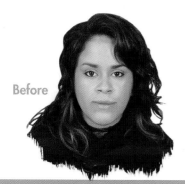

Before

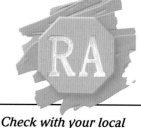

RA

OBJECTIVE

To use two or more levels of color to create bold and vibrant ribbons of color within a hairdesign, producing strong contrast to the natural haircolor.

Check with your local regulatory agency to see if the predisposition test is required 24-48 hours prior to the haircolor service.

TOOLS & MATERIALS

- Cloth and disposable towels
- Gloves
- Chemical apron
- Neck strip and cape/robe
- Color bowl and brush
- Applicator bottle

- Measuring cup
- Timer
- Hydrometer
- Color chart
- Shampoo and conditioner
- Protective cream

- Color stain remover
- Hair lightener
- Hydrogen peroxide
- Haircolor product
- Coloring combs
- Thermal tools

- Sectioning clips
- Cotton
- Liquid styling tools
- Haircoloring foils
- Client/guest record card

PROCEDURE

"The client/guest consultation is an important part of your professional service. Be sure to complete this step prior to each client/guest service you provide. Your successful retail sales and customer satisfaction rates depend upon it!"

RETAIL • RE-BOOK • REFERRAL

1. Cosmetologist sanitizes hands and station.
2. Set out service tools and materials.
3. Drape the client/guest in preparation for chemical service.
4. Perform scalp and hair analysis along with preliminary strand testing.

5. Follow procedure as shown and manufacturer's instructions.
6. Follow standard cleanup procedure.
7. Document client/guest record card.

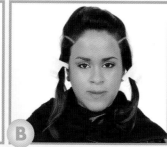

A Section hair according to desired end result **(side view).**

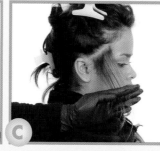

B Hair sectioning **(front view).** Refer to page 255 for foil pattern guide.

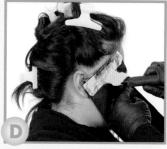

C Take ½ **inch to one inch (1.25 to 2.5 cm) diagonal partings using a slice technique.**

Place foil underneath subsection and **apply lightener to hair** starting at scalp area.

D

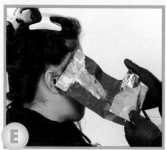

E Continue lightener application over entire subsection of hair.

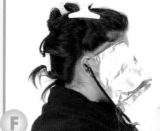

F Cover lightener with a single piece of foil. **Repeat steps C to F** on two more sliced partings and for three sliced partings on opposite side of head.

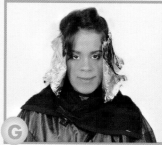

G Complete foiled sections. Process to desired lightness – perform a strand test.

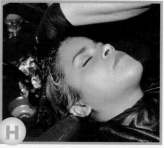

H Once desired lightness is achieved, remove foils, rinse and shampoo hair.

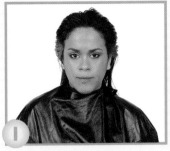

I Towel-dry and comb through hair.

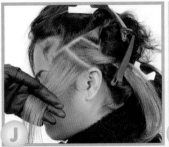

J **Subdivide sides into three subsections** using diagonal partings.

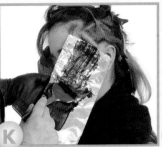

K **Apply three varying levels of red**, start with **the first level of red in the subsection** at the hairline.

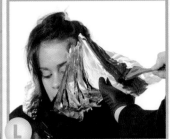

L Repeat step **K** with the **second level of red** in the second subsection.

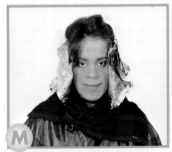

M Complete last subsection using the **third level of red. Repeat steps J to M** on opposite front section. Process following manufacturer's directions and/or results of strand test.

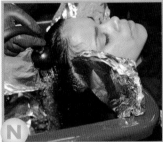

N Remove foils and rinse.

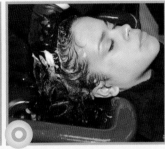

O Shampoo and condition the hair. Towel-dry and proceed with styling and finishing the hair.

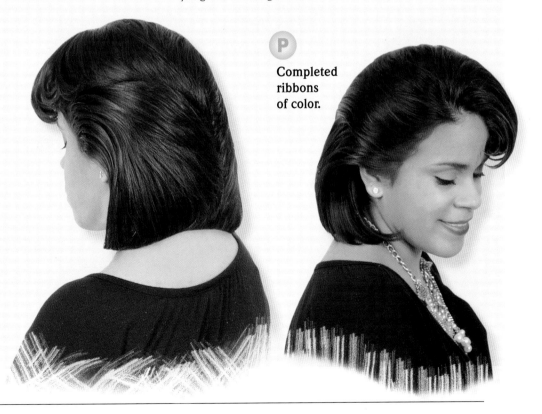

P Completed ribbons of color.

Before

Zone Coloring

OBJECTIVE

To create a dramatic, high-fashion hairdesign by placing two or more different levels of color in separate zones of the hair.

RA

Check with your local regulatory agency to see if the predisposition test is required 24-48 hours prior to the haircolor service.

TOOLS & MATERIALS

- Cloth and disposable towels
- Gloves
- Chemical apron
- Neck strip and cape/robe
- Color bowl and brush
- Applicator bottle

- Measuring cup
- Timer
- Hydrometer
- Color chart
- Shampoo and conditioner
- Protective cream

- Color stain remover
- Hair lightener
- Hydrogen peroxide
- Haircolor product (various colors)
- Coloring combs

- Thermal tools
- Sectioning clips
- Cotton
- Haircoloring foils
- Liquid styling tools
- Client/guest record card

PROCEDURE

"The client/guest consultation is an important part of your professional service. Be sure to complete this step prior to each client/guest service you provide. Your successful retail sales and customer satisfaction rates depend upon it!"

RETAIL · RE-BOOK · REFERRAL

1. Cosmetologist sanitizes hands and station.
2. Set out service tools and materials.
3. Drape the client/guest in preparation for a chemical service.
4. Perform a scalp and hair analysis along with preliminary strand testing.
5. Follow procedure as shown and manufacturer's instructions.
6. Follow standard cleanup procedure.
7. Document client/guest record card.

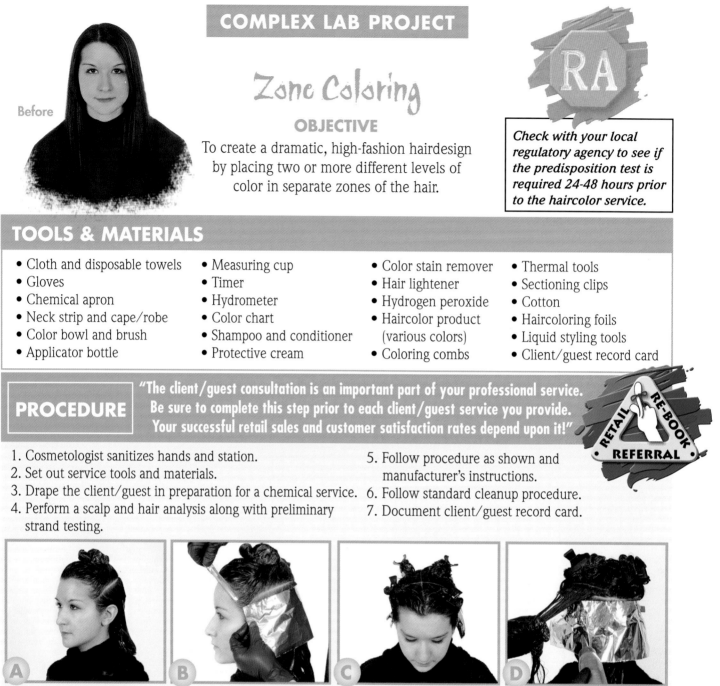

A Section hair according to hairdesign. **NOTE:** Model had existing highlighted hair so filler was placed on her hair prior to this zone color procedure.

B **Secure one piece of foil between zone one and two areas** to avoid overlapping of hair.

C Divide hair into four sections. Refer to page 256 for foil pattern guide.

D On **zone one,** take ½ to one inch (1.25 cm to 2.5 cm) **partings.**

E **Apply a low or high level color at scalp area.**

F Continue **applying color down strands to hair ends.**

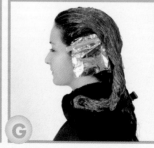

G Complete all four sections and turn foil up to cover top zone while coloring bottom zone.

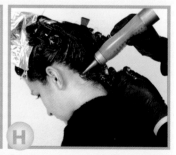

H On **zone two,** take ½ to one inch (1.25 cm to 2.5 cm) **partings.**

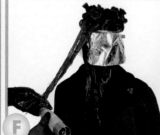

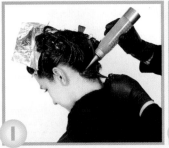

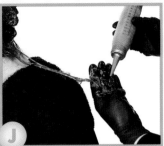

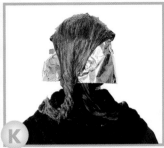

Apply an opposite **level of color** than what was applied on zone one – start at scalp area moving down over mid-strand.

Continue color application **to remaining hair.** Complete entire zone two area.

Completed color application of two zonal areas. Process and perform strand test. Remove foils, rinse, shampoo and condition the hair. Proceed with styling and finishing.

Completed zone coloring.

Base Dimensional Color (Star Pattern)

Before

OBJECTIVE

To blend the haircolor to the existing base level color by adding filler and to create a new design by combining both highlighting and lowlighting techniques on a pre-sectioned star pattern.

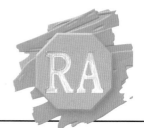
RA

Check with your local regulatory agency to see if the predisposition test is required 24-48 hours prior to the haircolor service.

TOOLS & MATERIALS

- Cloth and disposable towels
- Gloves
- Chemical apron
- Neck strip and cape/robe
- Color bowl and brush
- Applicator bottle

- Measuring cup
- Timer
- Hydrometer
- Color chart
- Shampoo and conditioner
- Protective cream

- Color stain remover
- Hair lightener
- Hydrogen peroxide
- Haircolor product (various colors)
- Coloring combs

- Sectioning clips
- Cotton
- Liquid styling tools
- Thermal tools
- Haircoloring foils
- Client record card/file

PROCEDURE

"The client/guest consultation is an important part of your professional service. Be sure to complete this step prior to each client/guest service you provide. Your successful retail sales and customer satisfaction rates depend upon it!"

RETAIL RE-BOOK REFERRAL

1. Cosmetologist sanitizes hands and station.
2. Set out service tools and materials.
3. Drape client/guest in preparation for chemical service.
4. Perform a scalp/hair analysis along with preliminary strand testing.
5. Follow procedure as shown and manufacturer's instructions.
6. Follow standard cleanup procedure.
7. Document client/guest record card.

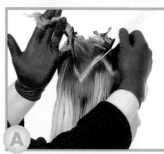

A Section hair on top of head into a star pattern.

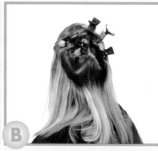

B Complete sectioned star pattern. Refer to page 257 for foil pattern guide.

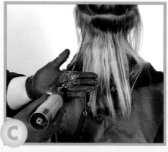

C Take ½ to one inch (1.25 to 2.5 cm) partings, apply filler to the pre-lightened hair.

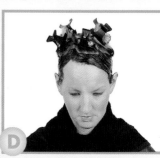

D Completed filler application (front view).

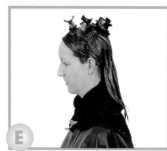

E Completed filler application (side view).

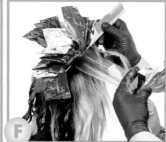

F Star Pattern Foiling Technique: For each triangle section of the star – slice ⅛ to ¼ inch (0.3 to 0.6 cm) parting of hair.

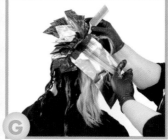

G Place foil underneath subsection hair.

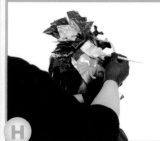

H Apply lightener from scalp to ends. NOTE: If hair has been lightened, **apply lightener to re-growth area ONLY.**

Base Dimensional Color (Star Pattern)

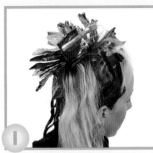

I Secure foil by folding in half and turning sides into center of packet.

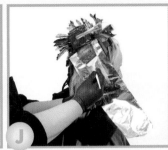

J Slice ⅛ to ¼ inch (0.3 to 0.6 cm) parting of hair and apply a low level color at scalp area.

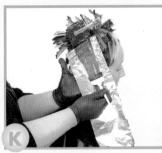

K Continue to apply color to remaining hair.

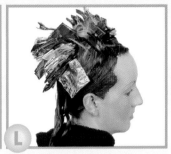

L A complete section consists of three foils with highlights and three with lowlights. Repeat pattern on remaining triangular sections.

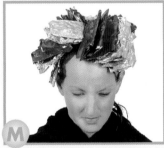

M Completed star pattern (front view). NOTE: Six foils in each triangular section.

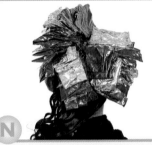

N Completed star pattern (back view). Process following manufacturer's directions and/or until desired shade is achieved.

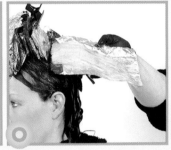

O Strand test to check for desired level of lightness.

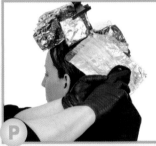

P When strand testing, remove lightener using ONLY a cloth towel.

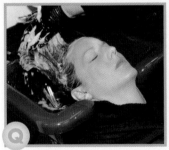

Q Remove foils, rinse, shampoo and condition the hair. Towel-dry and re-section.

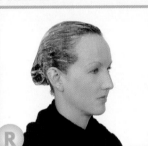

R Take ½ inch (1.25 cm) partings, apply a golden-blonde overlay of color from scalp to ends. Process, strand test for color development – rinse, shampoo and condition hair.

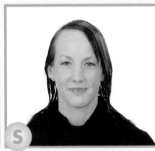

S Towel-dry and comb through hair. Proceed with styling and finishing.

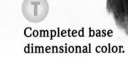

T Completed base dimensional color.

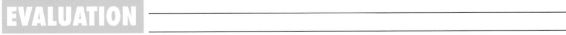

EVALUATION

GRADE STUDENT'S NAME ID#

Chapter 7 • **ART OF DIMENSIONAL HAIRCOLORING** 249

LOWLIGHTING

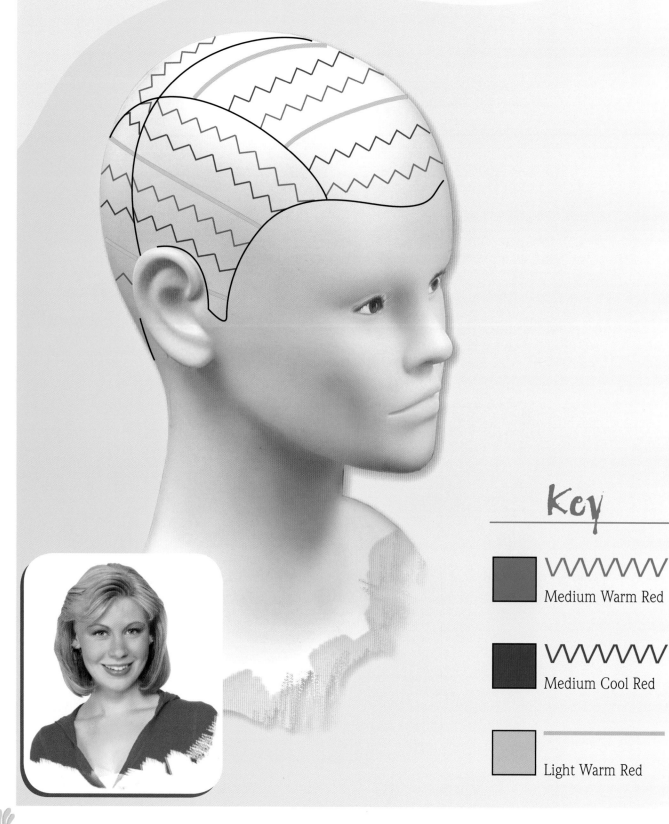

Key

■	\/\/\/\/ Medium Warm Red
■	\/\/\/\/ Medium Cool Red
■	—— Light Warm Red

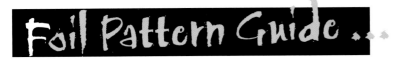
Foil Pattern Guide ...

HIGHLIGHTING (PARTIAL)

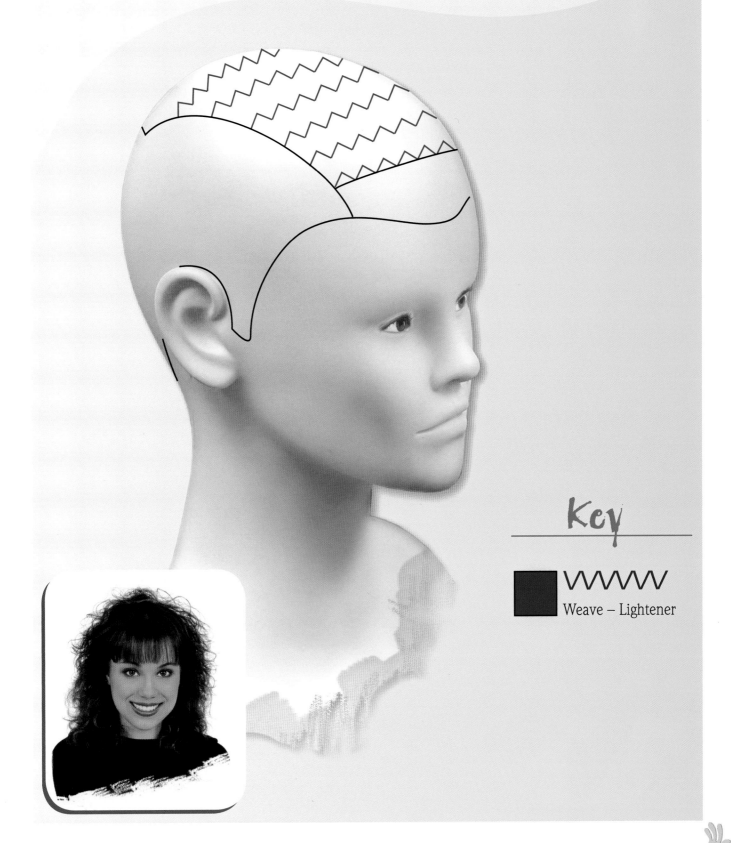

Key

VVVVV
Weave – Lightener

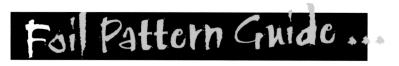

HIGHLIGHTING (FULL)

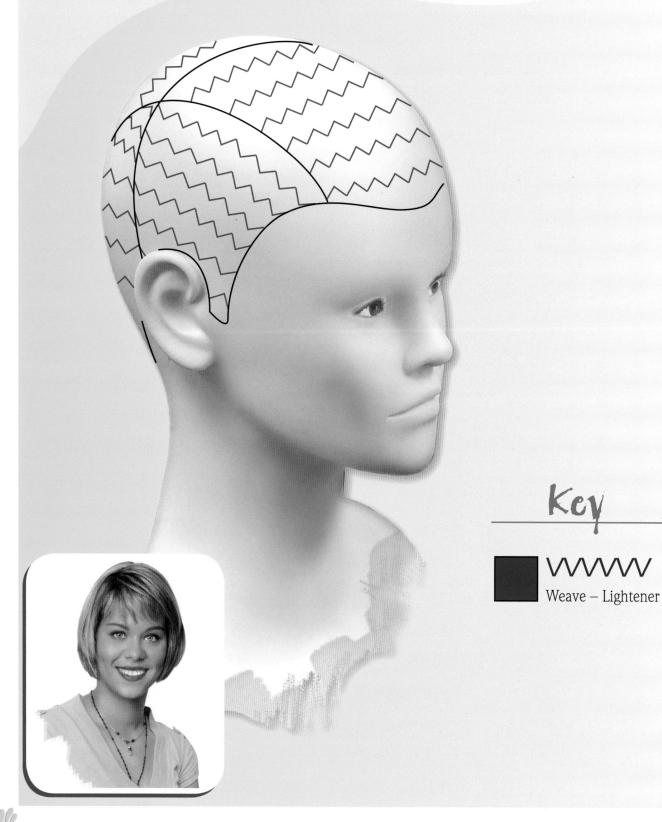

Key

⬛ VVVVV
Weave – Lightener

HIGHLIGHTING (CRISSCROSS)

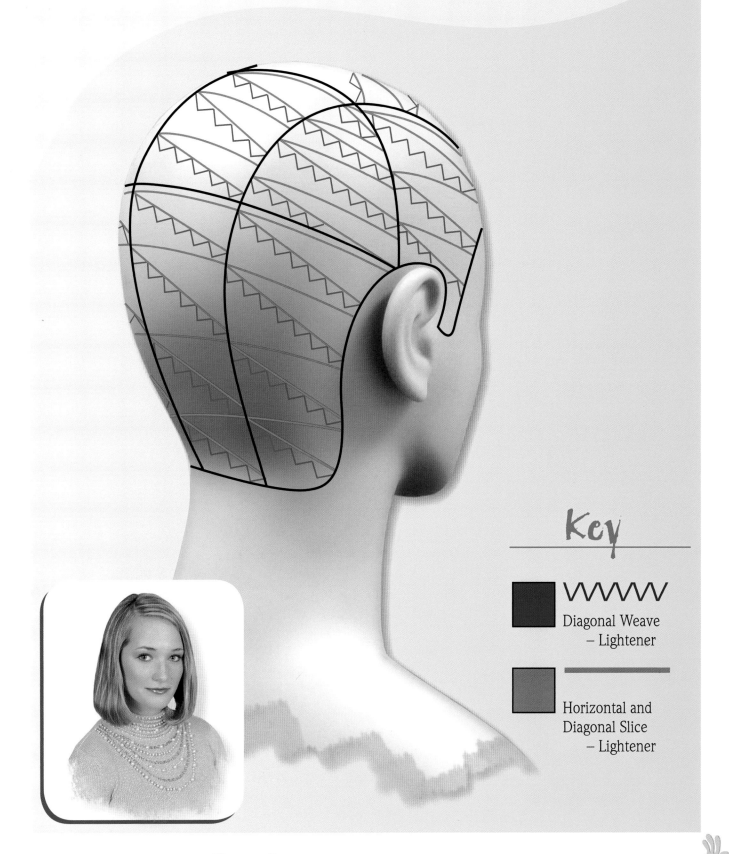

Key

⋀⋀⋀⋀⋀
Diagonal Weave
– Lightener

Horizontal and
Diagonal Slice
– Lightener

TONE-ON-TONE COLORING

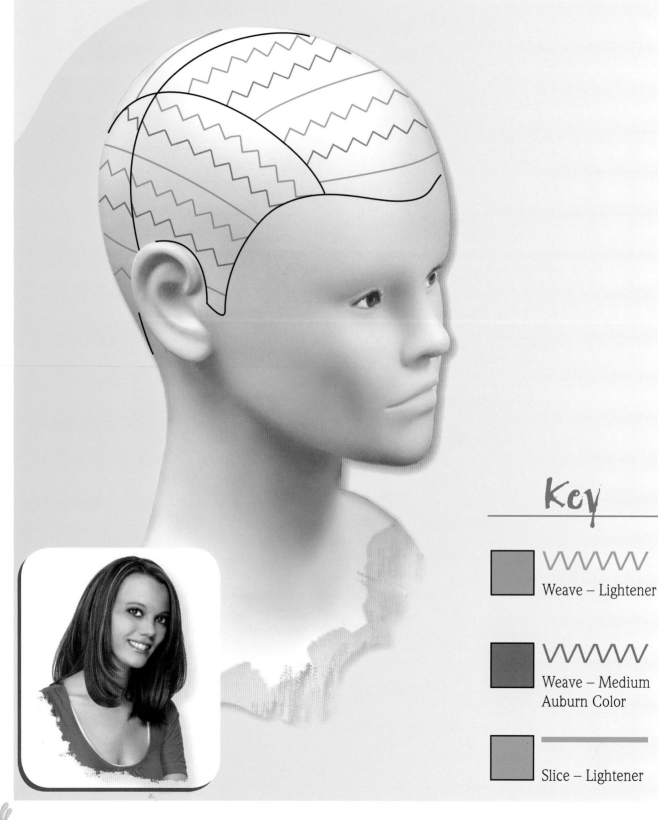

Key

◼ ∿∿∿∿∿ Weave – Lightener

◼ ∿∿∿∿∿ Weave – Medium Auburn Color

◼ ——— Slice – Lightener

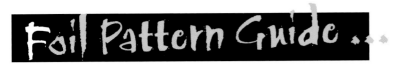

RIBBONS OF COLOR

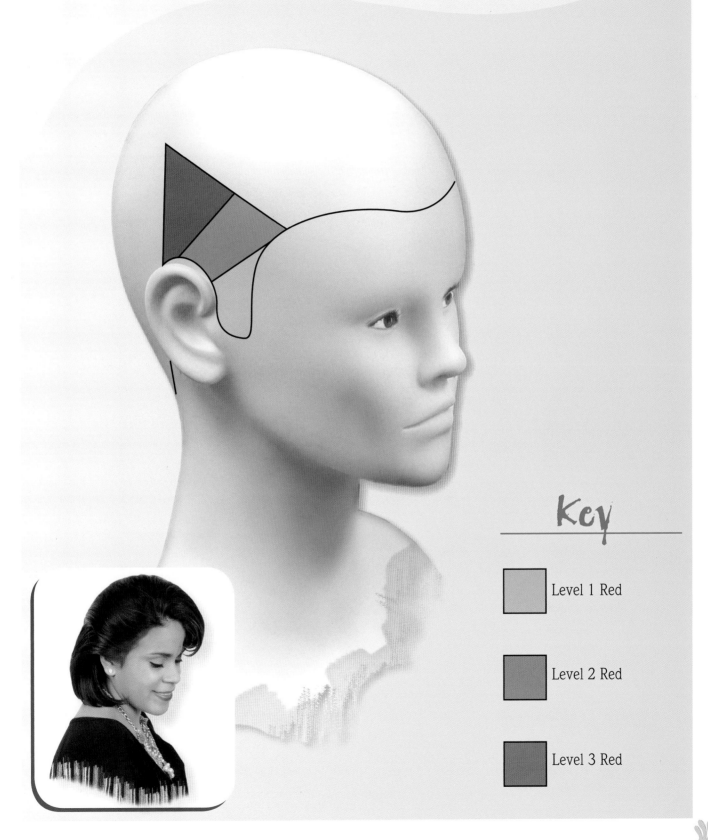

Key

Level 1 Red

Level 2 Red

Level 3 Red

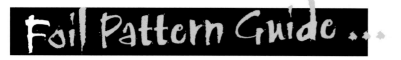
Foil Pattern Guide ...

ZONE COLORING

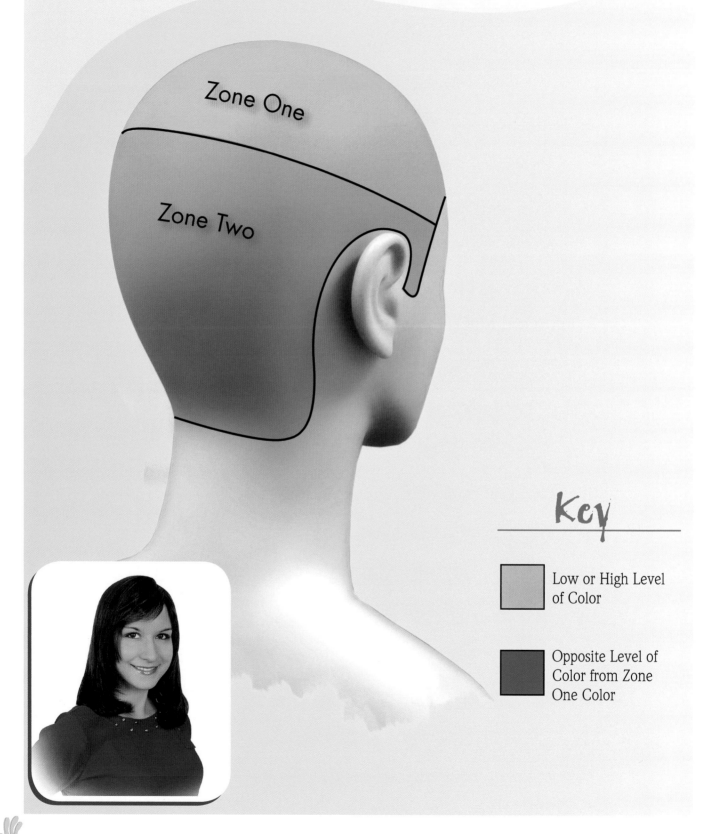

Zone One

Zone Two

Key

Low or High Level of Color

Opposite Level of Color from Zone One Color

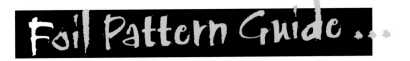
Foil Pattern Guide ...

BASE DIMENSIONAL COLOR (STAR PATTERN)

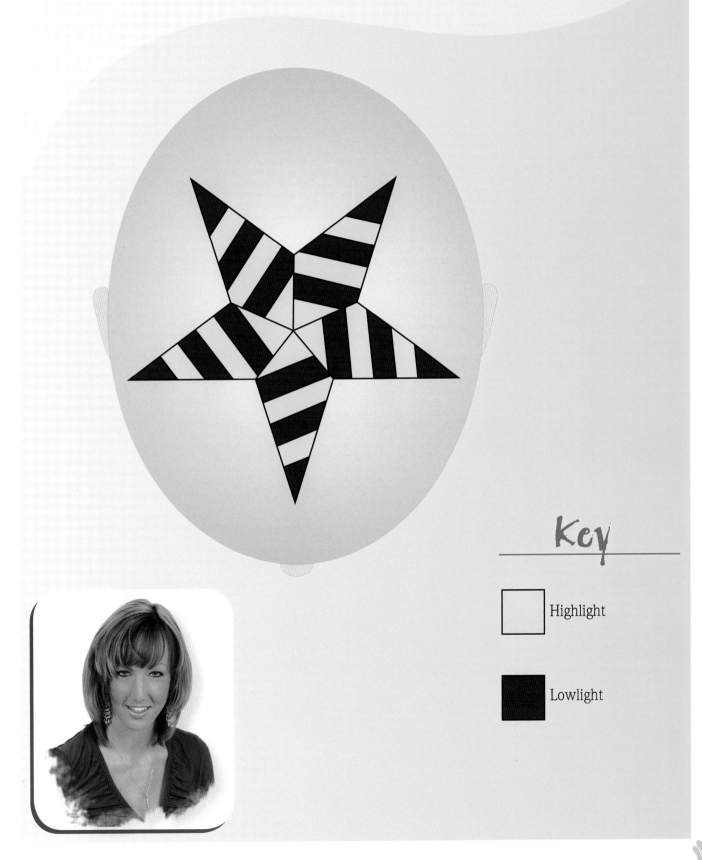

Key

Highlight

Lowlight

Become a color artist, not a color chartist!

by Randy Rick

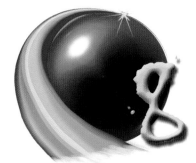

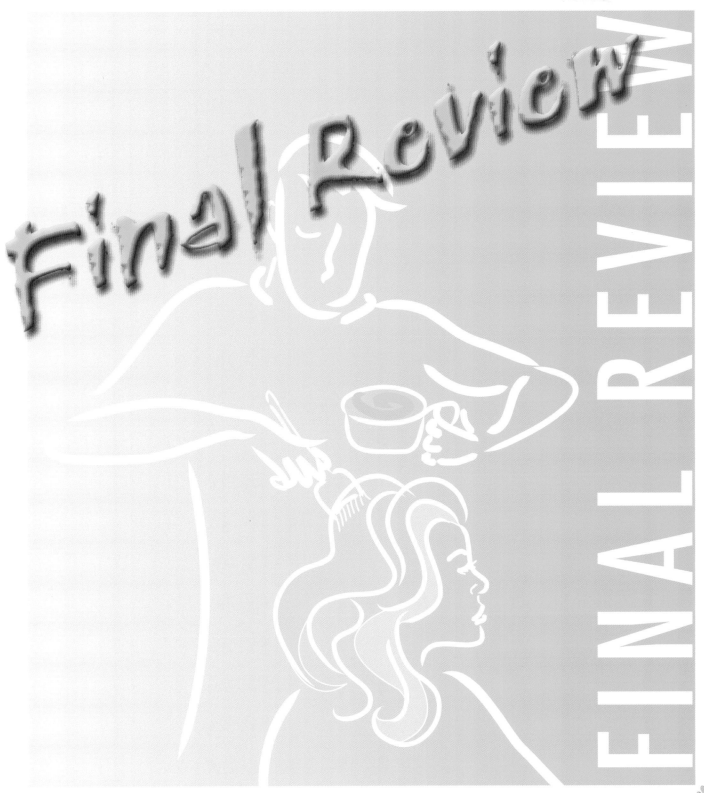

Final Review

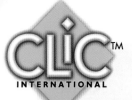
Haircoloring FINAL REVIEW QUESTIONS

FILL-IN-THE-BLANKS

A.	Ammonia
B.	Atoms
C.	Color Blindness
D.	Cuticle
E.	Eumelanin
F.	Gloves
G.	Haircolor Brush
H.	Haircolor Hook
I.	Hair Lightener
J.	Henna
K.	Light
L.	Liquid Haircolor
M.	Oxidation
N.	Pheomelanin
O.	Preliminary Strand Testing
P.	Protective Cream
Q.	Sulfur
R.	Temporary Haircolor
S.	Viscosity
T.	White Hair

1. _____ is used to pull hair through a haircolor cap.

2. _____ is an alkaline substance that emits a gaseous odor and is used in the manufacturing of haircolor.

3. _____ is used to apply color on the hair when taken from a color bowl.

4. _____ is a vegetable dye that is not always encouraged for use in a salon due to interference with other chemicals.

5. _____ are made up of protons, neutrons and electrons.

6. _____ is a form of energy that travels in invisible waves.

7. _____ is applying a pre-determined color formula to the hair to preview end color results.

8. _____ are used to protect the haircolorist's hands from stains and chemical sensitivity.

9. _____ is when a person is unable to visually differentiate between certain shades of color.

10. _____ is placed along the client/guest's hairline prior to haircolor application.

11. _____ is the tough, outer protective covering of the hair.

12. _____ provides better penetration of the cuticle than cream haircolor.

13. _____ produces brown to black pigments in the hair.

14. _____ coats the hair surface – covering only the cuticle.

15. _____ is the property of a fluid in which the flow is resisted; the thickness or heaviness of the liquid.

16. _____ is the chemical reaction that occurs when oxygen is released from a substance.

17. _____ has a total absence of pigment – no eumelanin or pheomelanin.

18. _____ pigmentation produces light eyes and creates yellow undertones in client/guest's hair when going lighter.

19. _____ produces yellow to red pigments in the hair.

20. _____ is sometimes referred to as bleach or decolorizer.

STUDENT'S NAME   DATE   GRADE

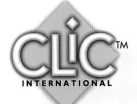

MULTIPLE CHOICE

1. Under what pH level range do haircolors and lighteners fall?
   A. acid   B. neutral   C. alkaline
2. What is the chemical symbol for hydrogen peroxide?
   A. H_2O_2 B. H_2O C. NH_3
3. Which of the following is NOT an example of dimensional haircoloring?
   A. corrective color   B. highlighting   C. lowlighting
4. Lead acetate is an ingredient used in what kind of haircoloring?
   A. vegetable dyes   B. metallic dyes   C. permanent color
5. High volumes of hydrogen peroxide oxidize at what speed?
   A. slow   B. same as 10 volumes   C. quick
6. What size partings are used for permanent color application?
   A. ⅛ inch (0.3 cm)   B. ¼ inch (0.6 cm)   C. ½ inch (1.25 cm)
7. What layer of the hair produces melanin?
   A. cuticle   B. cortex   C. medulla
8. What is one of the main and most important skills of a client/guest consultation?
   A. talking   B. listening   C. laughing
9. Which tool is used to measure the volumes of hydrogen peroxide?
   A. hydrometer   B. color key   C. applicator bottle
10. Temporary haircolor creates what kind of change to the hair?
    A. physical   B. chemical   C. permanent
11. What is the pH of distilled water?
    A. 3   B. 5.5   C. 7
12. What is the number of decolorization stages?
    A. seven   B. eight   C. nine
13. Which of the following is NOT considered a standard haircolor family or series?
    A. A-Ash   B. G-Gold   C. B-Black
14. What is the patch test reaction called when a client/guest cannot receive the haircolor?
    A. negative   B. neutral   C. positive
15. Which color is NOT part of the Visible Spectrum of Color?
    A. blue   B. white   C. indigo
16. What undertones are present in the client/guest with a natural level ranging from 1 to 3?
    A. red   B. gold   C. yellow
17. What type of shampoo is recommended when cleansing hair with artificial haircolor?
    A. acid-balanced   B. clarifying   C. medicated
18. Which haircolor service creates NO line of demarcation?
    A. permanent   B. semi-permanent   C. hair lightening
19. Which alkalizing agent is used in the manufacturing of haircolors or lighteners that has little to no odor?
    A. ammonia   B. hydrogen peroxide   C. alkanolamines
20. Which category of haircolor consists of both large and small direct dye molecules?
    A. temporary   B. semi-permanent   C. demi-permanent

STUDENT'S NAME   DATE   GRADE

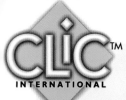

Haircoloring FINAL REVIEW QUESTIONS

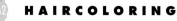

FILL-IN-THE-BLANKS

A.	Allergy
B.	Anagen
C.	Brown Color
D.	Cap and Hook Method
E.	Color Therapy
F.	Complementary Colors
G.	Diffuse
H.	Filler
I.	Fluorescent Lighting
J.	Free Hand Painting
K.	Haircolor Families
L.	Keratin
M.	Level
N.	Mascara
O.	Natural Light
P.	Natural Series
Q.	Neck Strips
R.	Permanent Haircolor
S.	Powder Lighteners
T.	Semi-Permanent Haircolor

1. _____ is an indoor light source that produces cool to drab tones on the skin and hair.

2. _____ is the strong, fibrous protein derived from the amino acids that make up the hair.

3. _____ is the ultimate source for viewing and determining a client/guest's natural haircolor level.

4. _____ or growing stage is when the hair continues to survive and grow.

5. _____ is a product that adds a missing primary color or equalizes the porosity of the cuticle.

6. _____ is when a body reacts with hypersensitivity to a normally harmless substance.

7. _____ simultaneously deposits artificial color and lightens natural haircolor.

8. _____ is not mixed with hydrogen peroxide – is referred to as a non-oxidative haircolor.

9. _____ is considered a form of a temporary haircolor.

10. _____ are wrapped around client/guest's neck to prevent skin-to-cape contact.

11. _____ is a natural therapeutic approach that uses color to affect our emotions and moods.

12. _____ is the degree of lightness or darkness of a color.

13. _____ decolorize the hair and are considered stronger than other lightening agents, and have a faster development time.

14. _____ are color hues and intensities on hair swatches, which are then separated into groups.

15. _____ are hair swatches colored with a blend of all three primary colors, but in unequal proportions.

16. _____ is pulling clean, dry hair through a perforated plastic or latex cap using a crochet hook.

17. _____ is the scattering of melanin or pigment in the hair allowing light reflection instead of absorption.

18. _____ are derived from mixing a primary and a secondary color that are situated opposite each other on the color wheel.

19. _____ is a combination of all three primaries, but in unequal proportions – three yellow, two red and one blue.

20. _____ is a technique that manually places haircolor or lightener on the hair surface.

STUDENT'S NAME   DATE   GRADE

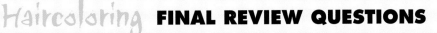

Haircoloring FINAL REVIEW QUESTIONS

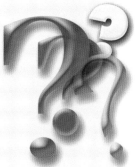

MULTIPLE CHOICE

1. What is created by mixing two primary colors together?
   A. secondary
   B. complementary
   C. neutral

2. Which color is found deepest within the hair shaft?
   A. blue
   B. red
   C. yellow

3. What do alkaline products do to the hair?
   A. swell
   B. contract
   C. harden

4. What area of the hair root supplies nourishment for continued hair fiber growth?
   A. follicle
   B. bulb
   C. dermal papilla

5. When lightener is applied to the hair, what happens to the melanin in the cortex layer?
   A. increases
   B. diffuses
   C. hardens

6. What is the average growth of hair per month?
   A. 1 inch (2.5 cm)
   B. ½ inch (1.25 cm)
   C. ¼ inch (0.6 cm)

7. Which type of haircolor penetrates the cuticle and partially into the cortex?
   A. temporary
   B. semi-permanent
   C. demi-permanent

8. The absorption of water/liquid into the hair within a relative amount of time is referred to as?
   A. elasticity
   B. density
   C. porosity

9. What is the result when melanin production gradually declines in the cortex layer?
   A. gray hair
   B. dark hair
   C. red hair

10. Who discovered the connection between light and color with his famous prism experiment?
    A. Albert Einstein
    B. Sir Isaac Newton
    C. Democritus

11. Which type of haircolor remains in the hair until the next shampoo?
    A. temporary
    B. semi-permanent
    C. permanent

12. Red-orange is considered which principle of color?
    A. primary
    B. secondary
    C. tertiary

13. What is filled out before and after every haircoloring service?
    A. client/guest record card
    B. release statement
    C. questionnaire

14. Which product when pH tested is considered high in alkalinity?
    A. ammonia
    B. distilled water
    C. hydrogen peroxide

15. What size partings are used for semi-permanent color application?
    A. ¼ to ½ inch (0.6 to 1.25 cm)
    B. ⅛ inch (0.3 cm)
    C. ½ to 1 inch (0.6 to 2.5 cm)

16. What size partings are used for a lightening (decolorization) application?
    A. ½ inch (1.25 cm)
    B. ¼ inch (0.6 cm)
    C. ⅛ inch (0.3 cm)

17. Which category of haircolor needs no retouching?
    A. permanent
    B. demi-permanent
    C. temporary

18. Which primary color is located closest to the hair surface and is removed first?
    A. red
    B. blue
    C. yellow

19. How should hydrogen peroxide be safely stored?
    A. in a cool, dry and dark area
    B. on the workstation
    C. in a clean, warm area

20. The pH scale is designed logarithmically, meaning each number represents _____ in multiples of 10.
    A. an increase
    B. a decrease
    C. both an increase and decrease

STUDENT'S NAME   DATE   GRADE

CLIC™ INTERNATIONAL

Haircoloring FINAL REVIEW QUESTIONS

FILL-IN-THE-BLANKS

A. Aniline Derivative Tint

B. Applicator Bottle

C. Capes

D. Chromatic

E. Cortical Fibers

F. Deposit

G. Developer

H. Hair Root

I. Hair Shaft

J. Highlighting

K. Line of Demarcation

L. Molecule

M. New Growth

N. Paraphen-ylenediamine

O. Pre-Softening

P. Progressive or Metallic Dyes

Q. Resistant Porosity

R. Tyrosine

S. Volume

T. Zonal Technique

1. _____ is an oxidizing agent also known as hydrogen peroxide.

2. _____ is a dimensional haircoloring service that lightens selected pieces of hair.

3. _____ are used to cover the client/guest's clothing to protect from damage during all hair services.

4. _____ is used to hold and apply the color mixture to the hair.

5. _____ or percentage is the amount of oxygen gas released from hydrogen peroxide.

6. _____ is created when one or more atoms combine and retain their chemical and physical properties.

7. _____ is the term used for the entry of color molecules into the hair.

8. _____ is the area of the hair strand where retouch color is applied.

9. _____ is another term that refers to the seven colors that are derived from the spectrum of light.

10. _____ is the amino acid found in the melanocyte cell, which is located in the cortex layer of the hair.

11. _____ is a dark band on the hair that is a result of haircolor overlapping onto previously colored hair.

12. _____ is the term used for the portion of hair located below the skin or scalp.

13. _____ or para dyes are the colorless molecules that turn to a color once the oxidation process takes place.

14. _____ receives the haircolor and is the portion of hair that extends beyond the skin or scalp.

15. _____ is placing a product on resistant areas of the hair to initiate the process of opening the cuticle scales.

16. _____ consists of sectioned areas or patterns on the head where two or more colors are placed.

17. _____ occurs when the cuticle scales are lying flat, making the amount of liquid absorbed minimal.

18. _____ creates a slow progression of color through repeated color applications.

19. _____ are grouped together to produce the cortex.

20. _____ or commonly known as permanent color, is made up of small colorless molecules.

STUDENT'S NAME   DATE   GRADE

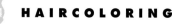
HAIRCOLORING

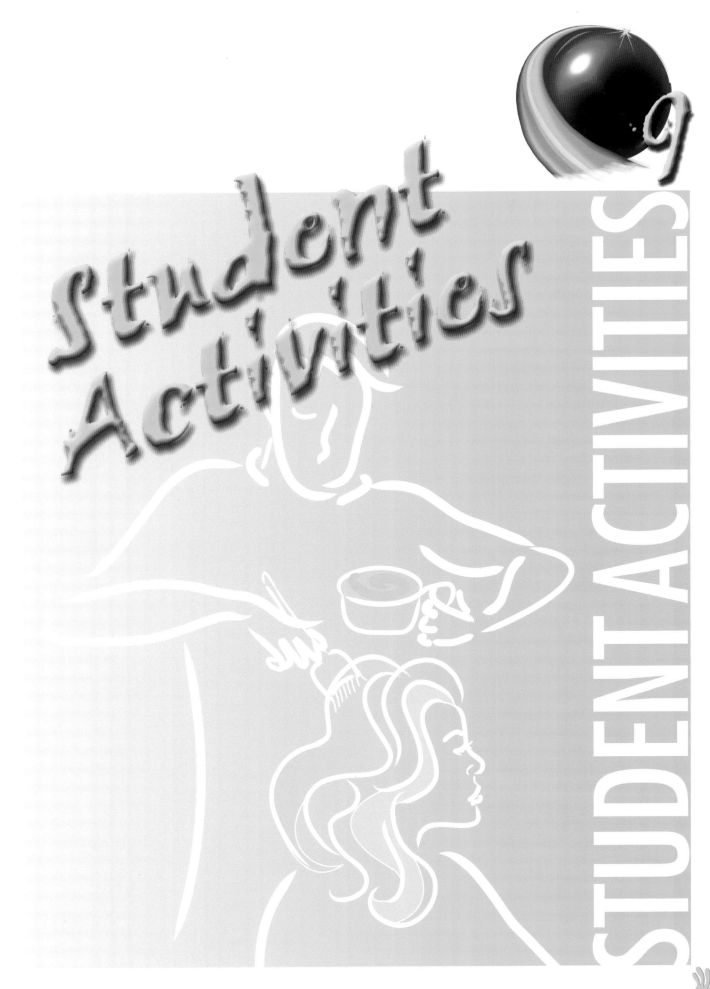

Student Activities

STUDENT ACTIVITIES

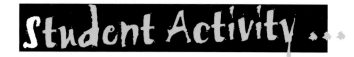
Directions: Paint or color in the primary colors. Mix the two primaries to find the secondary color. Paint or color in the secondary color and write the name.

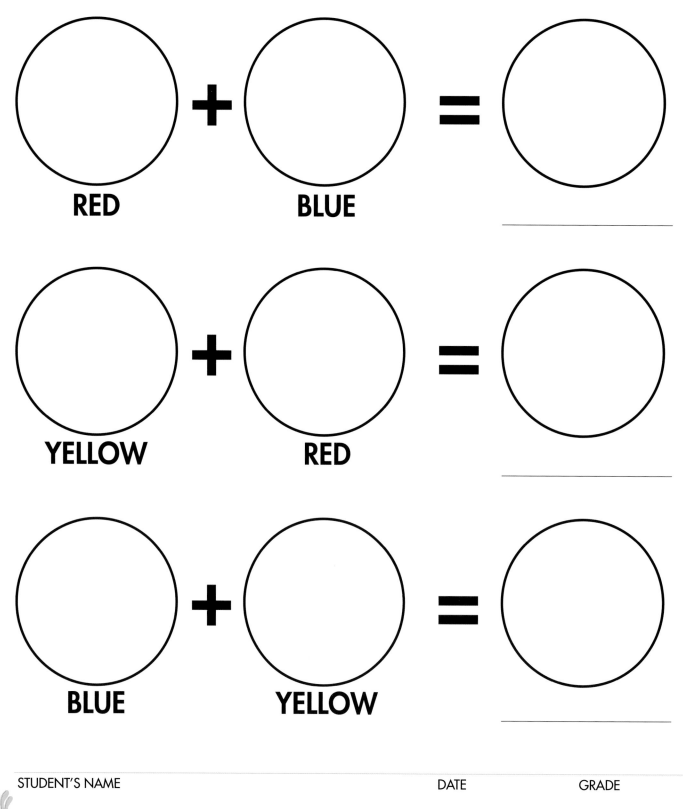

RED + BLUE =

YELLOW + RED =

BLUE + YELLOW =

Color Wheel Worksheet

Directions: Paint or color the three primary colors. Mix the two primary colors to create the secondary colors and place in appropriate areas of the color wheel. Mix the primary and secondary colors to create the tertiary colors and place in appropriate areas of the color wheel. Label each segment of the wheel with the name of the color represented.

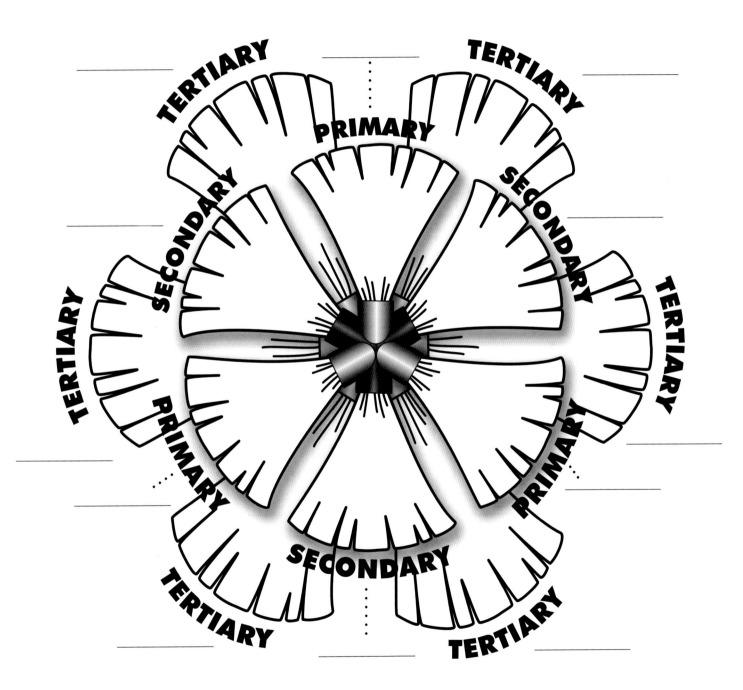

STUDENT'S NAME   DATE   GRADE

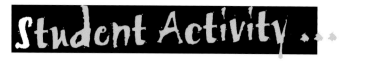

Student Activity

Directions: Based on the illustration, match the letter corresponding to each part of the hair structure to the correct name below.

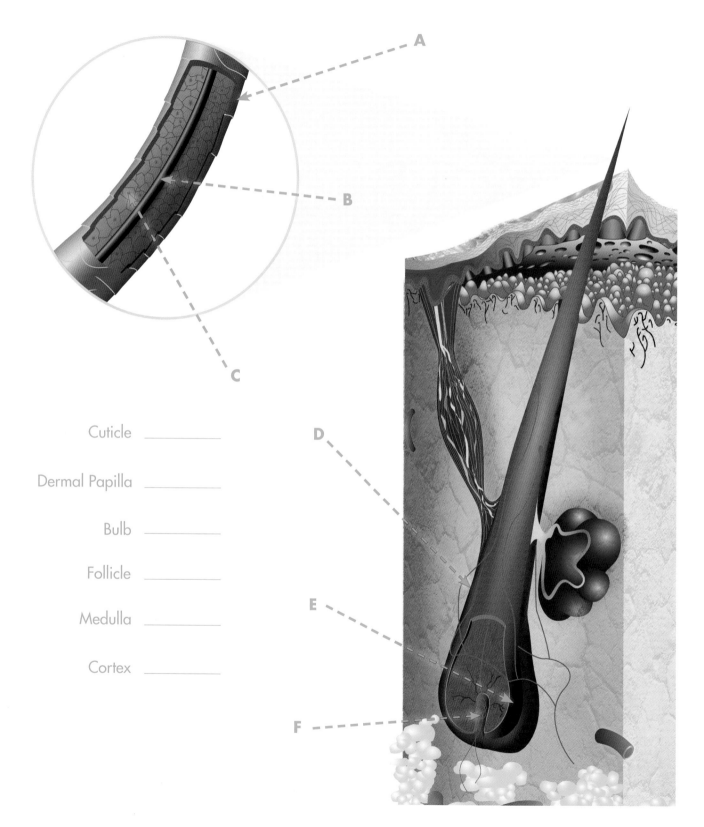

Cuticle _____

Dermal Papilla _____

Bulb _____

Follicle _____

Medulla _____

Cortex _____

Oxidative Haircolor Chart...

Make your own Oxidative Haircolor Chart using wefts of hair you color yourself.
After coloring each weft, attach it to the appropriate frame on the chart provided.

Color Series Name _____

Cut Slit ✂   Cut Slit ✂   Cut Slit ✂   Cut Slit ✂   Cut Slit ✂

Natural Level: _____   Natural Level: _____   Natural Level: _____   Natural Level: _____   Natural Level: _____
Color Formula: _____   Color Formula: _____   Color Formula: _____   Color Formula: _____   Color Formula: _____
Time: _____   Time: _____   Time: _____   Time: _____   Time: _____
Results: _____   Results: _____   Results: _____   Results: _____   Results: _____

Cut Slit ✂   Cut Slit ✂   Cut Slit ✂   Cut Slit ✂   Cut Slit ✂

Natural Level: _____   Natural Level: _____   Natural Level: _____   Natural Level: _____   Natural Level: _____
Color Formula: _____   Color Formula: _____   Color Formula: _____   Color Formula: _____   Color Formula: _____
Time: _____   Time: _____   Time: _____   Time: _____   Time: _____
Results: _____   Results: _____   Results: _____   Results: _____   Results: _____

STUDENT'S NAME _____   DATE _____   GRADE _____

Oxidative Haircolor Chart...

Tape Hair
Weft Here ✂

Tape Hair
Weft Here ✂

Tape Hair
Weft Here ✂

Tape Hair
Weft Here ✂

Tape Hair
Weft Here ✂

Tape Hair
Weft Here ✂

Tape Hair
Weft Here ✂

Tape Hair
Weft Here ✂

Tape Hair
Weft Here ✂

Tape Hair
Weft Here ✂

STUDENT'S NAME   DATE   GRADE

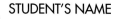

HAIRCOLORING

Oxidative Haircolor Chart

Make your own Oxidative Haircolor Chart using wefts of hair you color yourself.
After coloring each weft, attach it to the appropriate frame on the chart provided.

_____

Color Series Name

Cut Slit ✂   Cut Slit ✂   Cut Slit ✂   Cut Slit ✂   Cut Slit ✂

Natural Level: _____   Natural Level: _____   Natural Level: _____   Natural Level: _____   Natural Level: _____

Color Formula: _____   Color Formula: _____   Color Formula: _____   Color Formula: _____   Color Formula: _____

Time: _____   Time: _____   Time: _____   Time: _____   Time: _____

Results: _____   Results: _____   Results: _____   Results: _____   Results: _____

Cut Slit ✂   Cut Slit ✂   Cut Slit ✂   Cut Slit ✂   Cut Slit ✂

Natural Level: _____   Natural Level: _____   Natural Level: _____   Natural Level: _____   Natural Level: _____

Color Formula: _____   Color Formula: _____   Color Formula: _____   Color Formula: _____   Color Formula: _____

Time: _____   Time: _____   Time: _____   Time: _____   Time: _____

Results: _____   Results: _____   Results: _____   Results: _____   Results: _____

STUDENT'S NAME   DATE   GRADE

Chapter 9 • **STUDENT ACTIVITIES**

Oxidative Haircolor Chart...

Tape Hair Weft Here ✂   Tape Hair Weft Here ✂   Tape Hair Weft Here ✂   Tape Hair Weft Here ✂   Tape Hair Weft Here ✂

Tape Hair Weft Here ✂   Tape Hair Weft Here ✂   Tape Hair Weft Here ✂   Tape Hair Weft Here ✂   Tape Hair Weft Here ✂

STUDENT'S NAME   DATE   GRADE

Stages of Decolorization ...

Lighten and process six wefts to match each of the decolorization (brown, red, red-gold, gold, yellow and pale yellow) stages, leaving one weft untouched to represent the black stage. Rinse, dry and attach each weft to its appropriate frame on the chart provided.

Cut Slit ✂

Cut Slit ✂

Cut Slit ✂

Cut Slit ✂

Natural Level: _____

Natural Level: _____
Lightener Formula: _____
Time: _____
Stage: Brown_____

Natural Level: _____
Lightener Formula: _____
Time: _____
Stage: Red_____

Natural Level: _____
Lightener Formula: _____
Time: _____
Stage: Red-Gold_____

Cut Slit ✂

Cut Slit ✂

Cut Slit ✂

Natural Level: _____
Lightener Formula: _____
Time: _____
Stage: Gold_____

Natural Level: _____
Lightener Formula: _____
Time: _____
Stage: Yellow_____

Natural Level: _____
Lightener Formula: _____
Time: _____
Stage: Pale Yellow____

STUDENT'S NAME   DATE   GRADE

Stages of Declorization ...

Tape Hair
Weft Here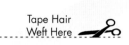

Tape Hair
Weft Here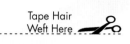

Tape Hair
Weft Here

Tape Hair
Weft Here

Tape Hair
Weft Here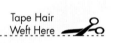

Tape Hair
Weft Here

Tape Hair
Weft Here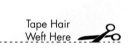

STUDENT'S NAME   DATE   GRADE

Haircolor and Decolorization Chart...

Optional: Place each weft worksheet inside individual acetate sleeves to protect the hair wefts and insert into a three-ring binder. Refer to this personal color chart when formulating color.

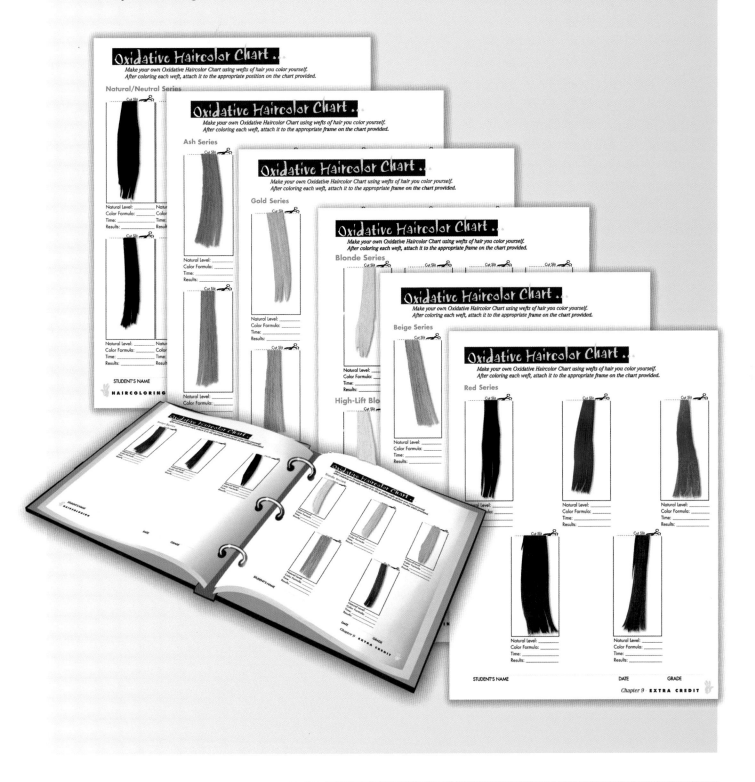

STUDENT'S NAME   DATE   GRADE

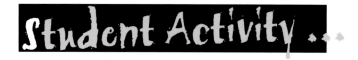

Client/Guest Color Card

Client/Guest Name _____

Address _____

Phone _____ Fax _____ E-Mail _____

Birthday (month/day)_____ Anniversary _____

Predisposition Test Results _____ Positive _____ Negative _____

Administered _____ Examined _____

Color Artist's Name _____

Client/Guest Haircolor Level _____ Percentage of Gray _____
                            Natural   Desired

Condition of Hair _____

Custom Formulation_____

Timing _____
          Scalp   Mid-Strand   Hair Ends

First Time Color Results and Adjustments _____

Retouch Color Formulation _____

Retouch Results and Adjustments _____

SERVICE DATE

SERVICE PRICE

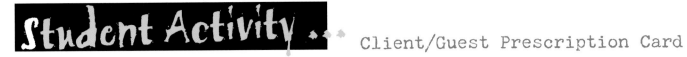 **Client/Guest Prescription Card**

Home Maintenance for Client/Guest's Hair

Client/Guest Name _____

Stylist's Name _____

Shampoo _____

_____

_____

Conditioner _____

_____

_____

Styling Aids _____

_____

_____

Finishing Products _____

_____

_____

Next Reservation in _____Weeks

Advanced Color Project...

Zones with Ribbons of Color

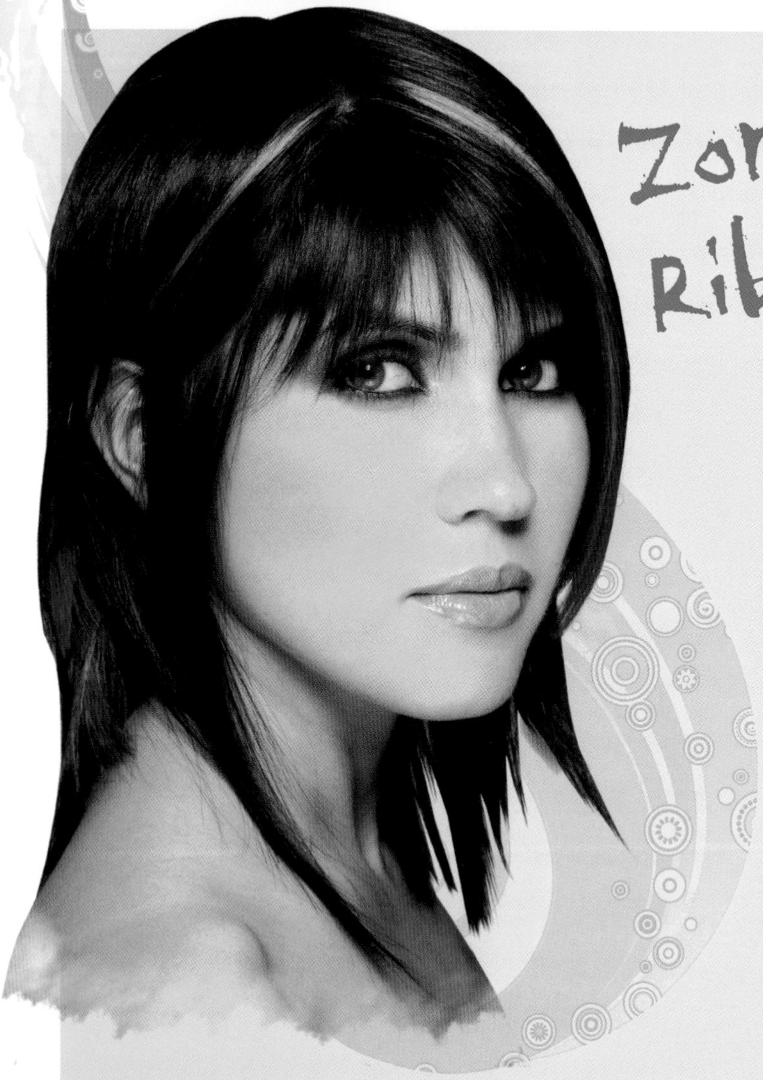

The combination of **zones with ribbons of color** is definitely an eye catcher! Each section on the head has an **array of different colored zones, along with the contrasting ribbons of color to create a true fashion statement.** The front view of the hairdesign will show the contrasting ribbon color along the sides and through the back of the hairstyle. As the professional, wear the zones with ribbons of color in your own hair and see how many client/guests request this method of haircolor.

NOTES

STUDENT'S NAME DATE GRADE

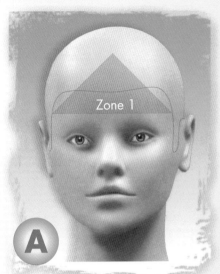

A

Part a triangle section along the frontal fringe area ... this will be **zone one.**

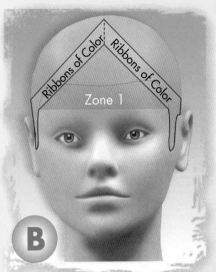

B

Part a ½ **to 1 inch (1.25 to 2.5 cm) subsection** along the back perimeter of triangle extending down to hairline at sides of head. **This subsection is used for the ribbon of color – wrap in foil to protect the hair.**

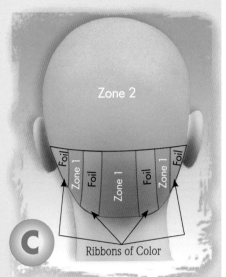

C

At back of head, below the occipital, create a section parted from middle of ear to ear down to the nape area. **Sub-divide two-½ to 1 inch (1.25 to 2.5 cm) subsections** on both sides of the center section. These four subsections are used for **ribbons of color** and the three remaining subsections will be referred to as **zone one.** Wrap the ribbons of color subsections in foil.

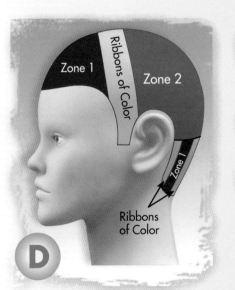

D

Apply a dark level of color on all zone one areas. Apply a medium level of color on entire zone two areas (refer to illustration). Process following manufacturer's instructions. Rinse, shampoo and condition, being careful not to touch the ribbon subsections.

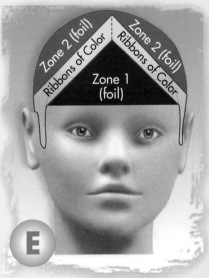

E

Apply lightener to all ribbon subsections, placing new foil around each subsection to protect the previously colored hair. Process to desired stage of decolorization determined from the preliminary strand test. Rinse, shampoo and towel dry hair.

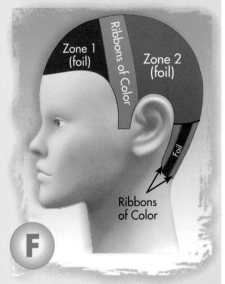

F

Apply a desired light level, fashion or vibrant color to the lightened hair, placing new foil around each subsection to protect the previously colored hair. Process and perform development strand test to determine color absorption. Once desired color is achieved, rinse, shampoo and condition hair. Style hair into finished hairdesign.

Sponge Spots

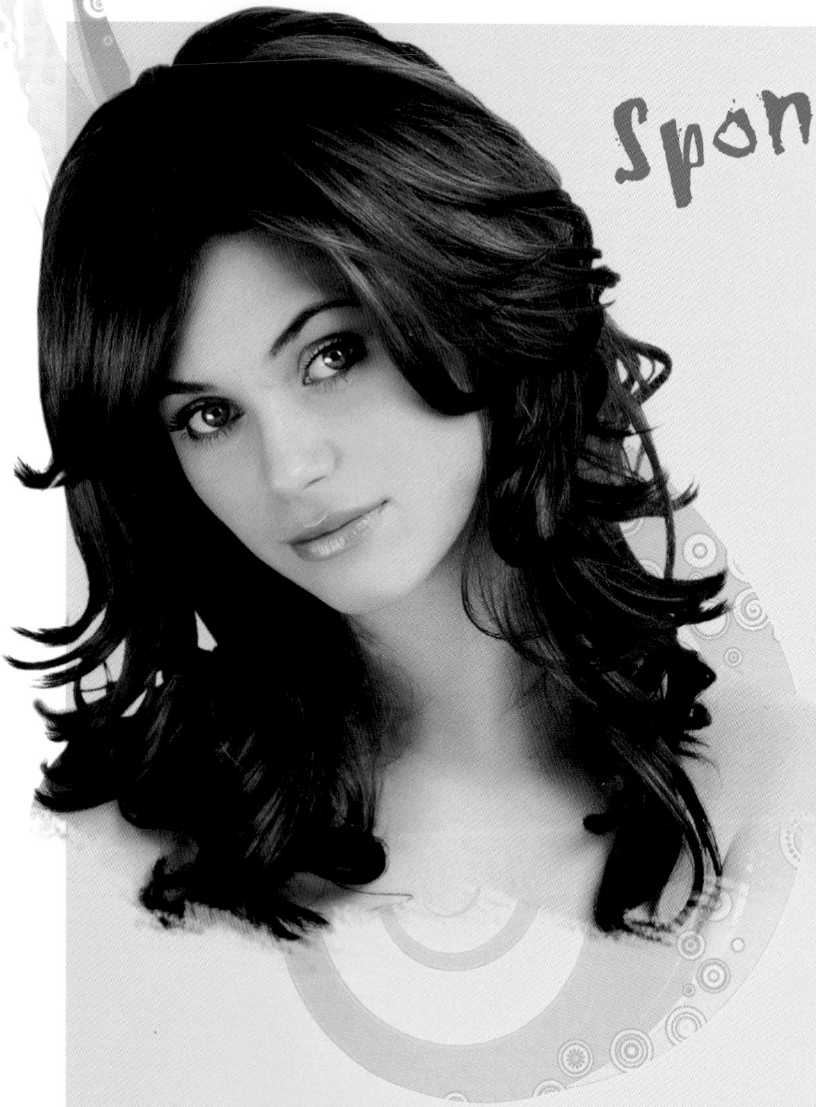

Sponge spots haircolor design is a free form painting technique, whereby the hair ends are touched with a **color that contrasts with the main overall color.** In this particular design, a **medium red-orange color** is applied to the hair as the overall (base) color and then a contrasting **dark color is sponged on the hair ends.** The **sponge application provides a less defined finish,** which is necessary to give this technique a more natural appearance.

NOTE: As an option, you may create the opposite contrasting effect by placing a dark level color as your base and then apply a medium to light color on the hair ends.

NOTES

STUDENT'S NAME DATE GRADE

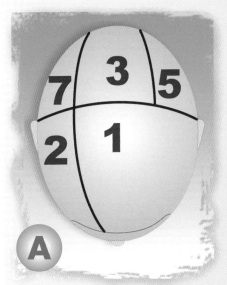

A

Once the overall (base) color application is completed, create a **vertical parting from hairline (inner corner of eye) to the vertical parting that is divided from ear to ear.** One section averages ⅔ in size and second section averages ⅓ in size.

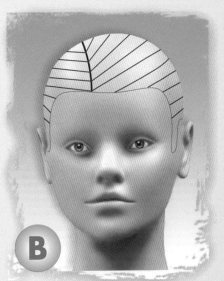

B

Starting at top of each section, create **diagonal partings** (45-degree angle) that eventually graduate to **horizontal partings.**

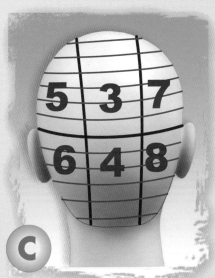

C

Create sections three through eight on back of head, starting with a center back panel and two side back panels. Divide the center and two side-back panels into six sections using an ear to ear horizontal parting. **Part 1 to 1½ inch (2.5 to 3. 81 cm) horizontal subsections** within each of the six sections.

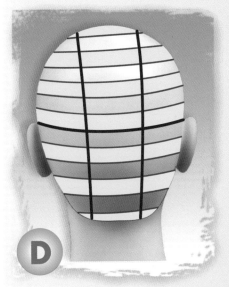

D

Start in nape area – every other subsection (yellow areas shown on illustration) receives the contrasting color ONLY on hair ends. Place subsection of hair on foil, **dip a small piece of sponge into color mixture and saturate 1 to 1½ inches (2.5 to 3.81 cm) of the hair ends ONLY in a free form pattern.**

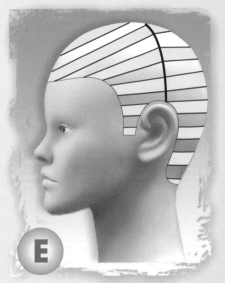

E

Repeat the same color application on the front subsections (refer to highlighted areas on illustration); begin at the ear area and move to the top sections. Complete entire head.

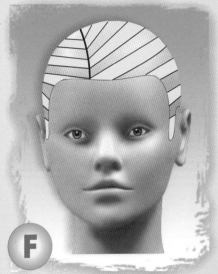

F

Process and perform development strand test to determine color absorption. Once desired color is achieved, rinse, shampoo and condition hair. Style hair into finished hairdesign.

Advanced Color Project ...

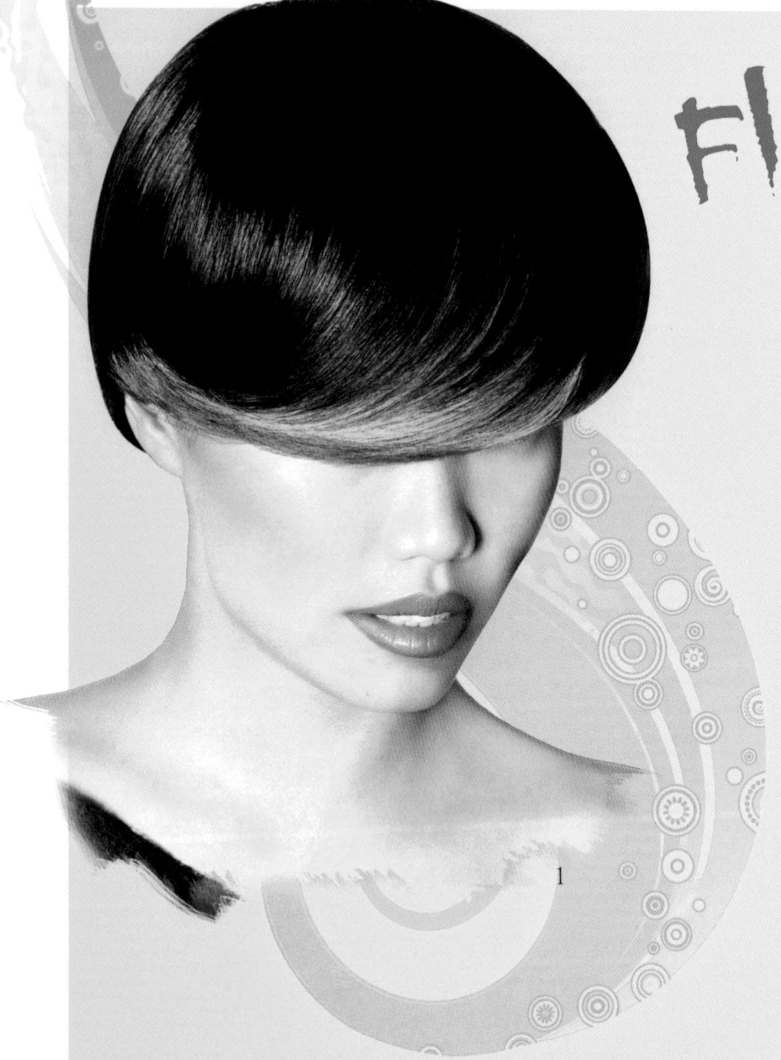

Flash Color

Flash haircoloring is an exciting, fun color technique that catches your eye and questions the admirer, "How did you do that?" In order to accomplish this color illusion, the **hair must be cut at a low elevation** – a maximum of 30 degrees or less will produce optimal results. To the viewer, **the hairstyle appears as having a subtle highlight along the outer perimeter of the design,** but when the hair is not in its natural fall distribution, a display of more color will appear to the observer.

NOTE: Hairdesigns cut to one length or in multiple layers are not recommended for this color technique, as it will not produce the true beauty of the flash color.

NOTES

STUDENT'S NAME DATE GRADE

...

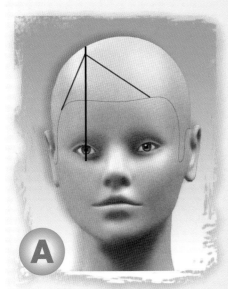

A

Divide a small vertical parting at the hairline using the center of eye as the point of reference. Begin the **first triangle at this parting,** extending the triangle to the corner of the opposite eye.

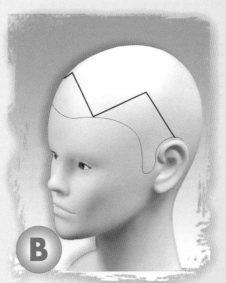

B

Continue to part a **wide triangle** along hairline on **side of hairdesign.**

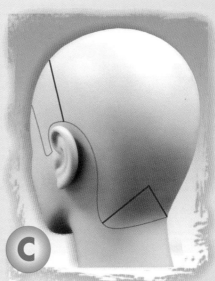

C

Divide a **wide triangle only at nape hairline.** Do not part a triangle behind the ears – this hair will receive the dark level color application.

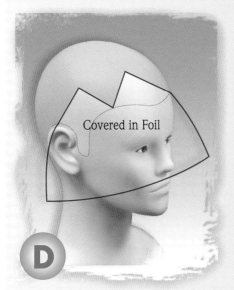

D

Continue to part a **wide triangle** along the hairline on **opposite side of hairdesign. Enclose perimeter triangles in foil** to protect hair from the color application on the interior area of design.

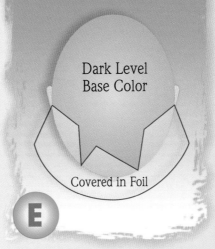

Dark Level Base Color

Covered in Foil

E

Apply a dark level (base) color to hair above the perimeter triangles (interior of design). Process and perform development strand test to determine color absorption. Once desired color is achieved, rinse, shampoo and condition hair. Towel dry hair and **place foil on hair to protect from the lightener application** on perimeter (triangle) hair.

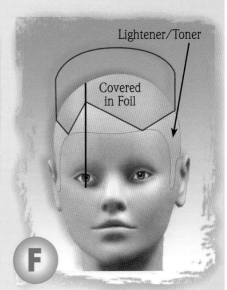

Lightener/Toner

Covered in Foil

F

Apply lightener to hair along perimeter and enclose in foil. Process and perform development strand test to determine decolorization stage. Once desired stage is reached, rinse, shampoo and towel dry hair. **Apply a toner to the lightened hair.** Process, strand test, rinse, shampoo and condition hair. Style hair into finished hairdesign.

Advanced Color Project ...

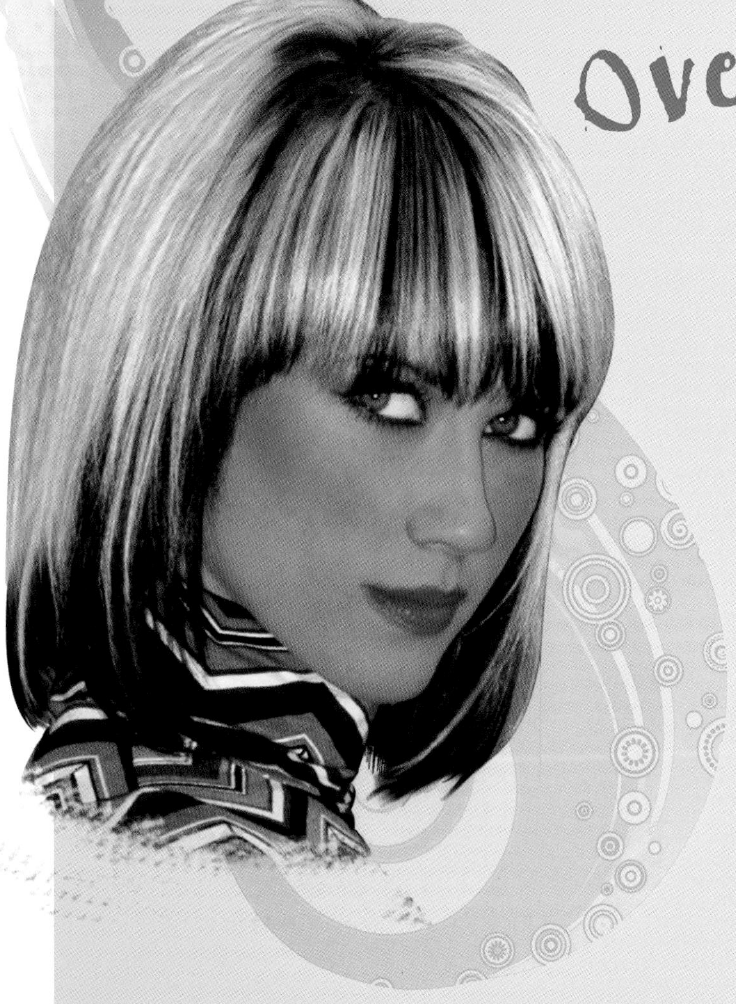

Overlays of Color

Overlays of color reveal an expression of the artist's imagination – each direction the hair is combed **displays an array of colors.** Think of a **kaleidoscope** – as you are looking through the tube and moving the dial, a **multiple arrangement of colors will appear.** It will show various patterns of shapes and colors with each turn ... the same applies with the overlays of color.

Add the overlays of color to your service list ... it can be your approach to keeping ahead of the competition. For the client/ guest who is open to new, fashionable color techniques, this is the color method of choice. Always remember, you are an image of your own work – market these creative color techniques by displaying them on yourself!

NOTES

STUDENT'S NAME DATE GRADE

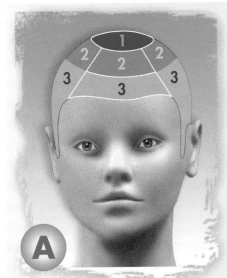

A

Part a triangle section along the frontal fringe area ...this will be **zone three, along with lower occipital, nape, lower side and sideburns.** Subsection the triangle into two more zones – zones two and one. **Zone two will encompass mid-occipital and sides of head. Zone one is directly on top of the head in an enclosed circle.**

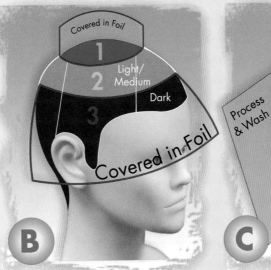

B

Cover zone one in foil to protect the hair from color application on zones two and three. **Apply a dark level of color to zone three. Place foil along top parting to cover zone three. Apply a medium to light level of color to zone two** (refer to illustration).

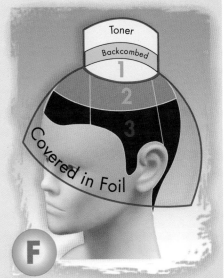

C

Process zones three and two following manufacturer's instructions. Rinse, shampoo, condition and towel dry hair of zones three and two.

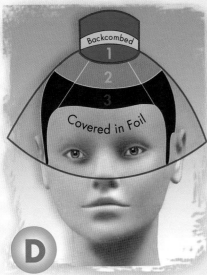

D

Place foil on top of previously colored hair and lightly backcomb zone one hair – create a two inch (5 cm) cushion of hair (refer to illustration).

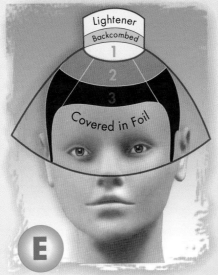

E

Apply lightener on mid-strand to hair ends – do not apply lightener to the two inch (5 cm) cushion of hair. Process to desired stage of decolorization determined from the preliminary strand test. Rinse, shampoo and towel dry hair.

F

Reapply foil on previously colored hair to protect from zone one color application. **Lightly backcomb zone one hair to create a two inch (5 cm) cushion of hair and apply a toner color to only the lightened hair – enclose in foil.** Process and perform development strand test to determine color absorption. Once desired color is achieved, rinse, shampoo and condition hair. Style hair into finished hairdesign.

Haircoloring Portfolio ...

The following Student Activity pages will help you create your own haircoloring portfolio.

- Find pictures in magazines showing variations of the haircoloring techniques pictured on the following pages.

- Attach your pictures in the open frames.

- Remove the pages and place in a three-ring binder.

- Have your first portfolio ready to show the client/guest(s), illustrating the various haircoloring designs offered. Update your portfolio as you learn more complex haircoloring techniques.

Optional: As you move from your student portfolio to a professional portfolio, you will showcase the haircoloring designs you have created. Purchase a portfolio case with individual acetate sleeves and insert 4" x 6" or 8" x 10" photographs of your haircoloring designs.

Haircoloring Portfolio...

Find examples of textures in different color levels.

LIGHT LEVELS

MEDIUM LEVELS

DARK LEVELS

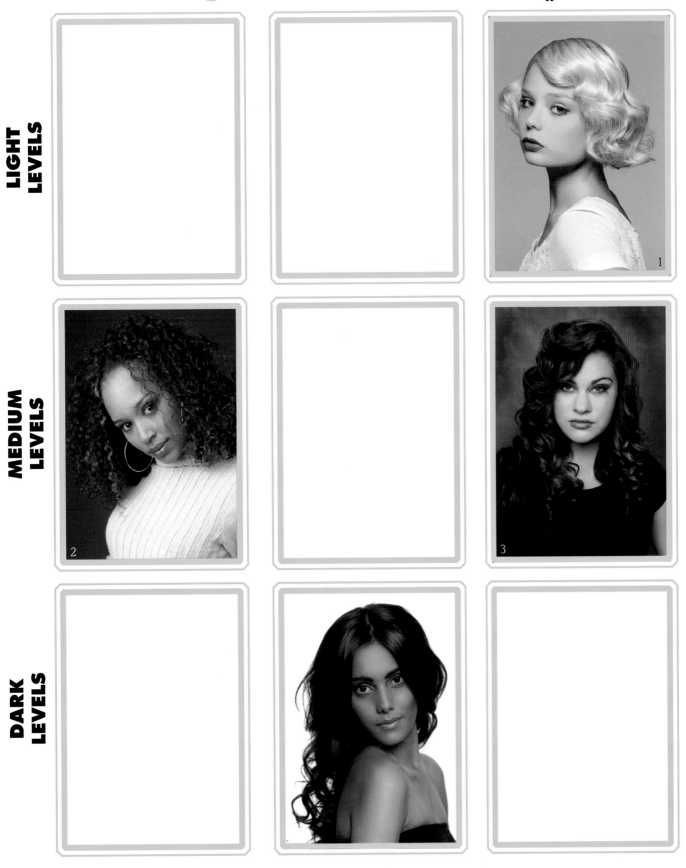

STUDENT'S NAME   DATE   GRADE

Haircoloring Portfolio ...

Find examples of high-lift blonde haircolors.

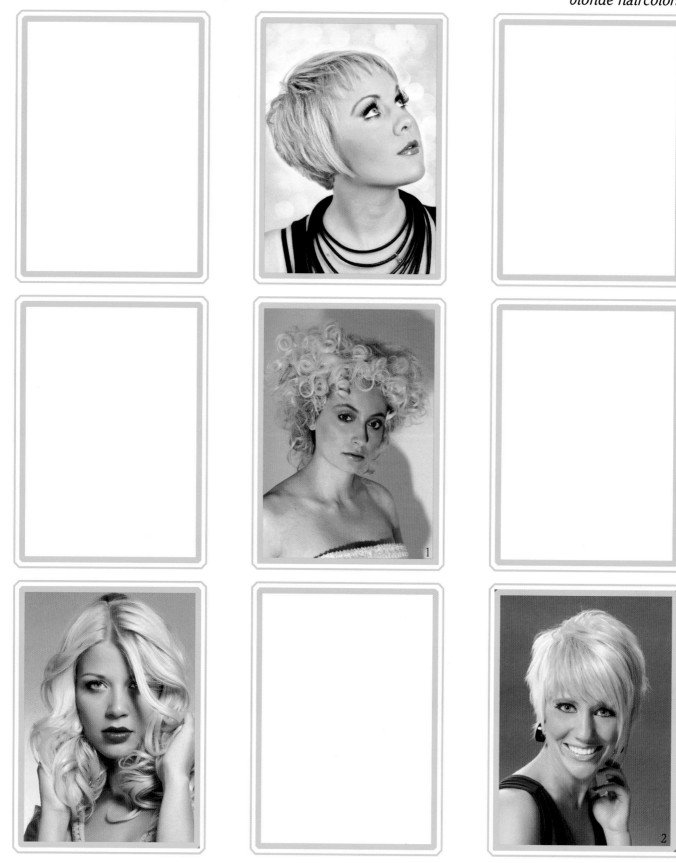

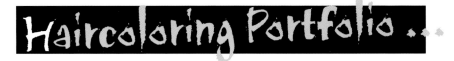

Haircoloring Portfolio ...

Find examples of highlights.

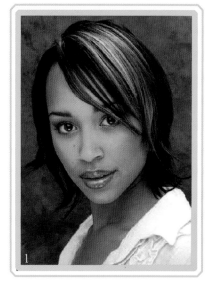

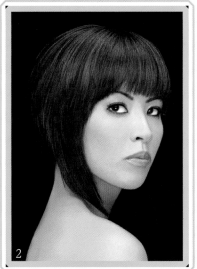

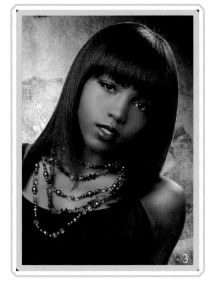

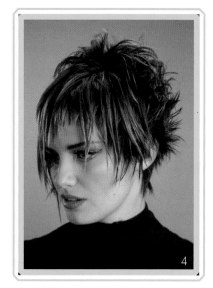

STUDENT'S NAME

DATE

GRADE

Haircoloring Portfolio ...

Find examples of lowlights.

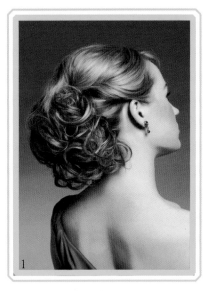

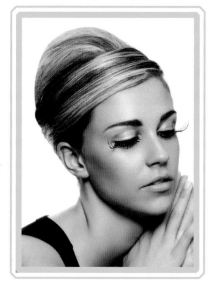

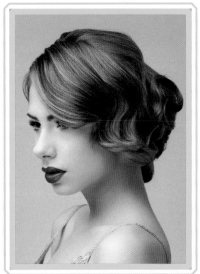

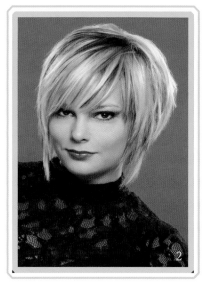

STUDENT'S NAME   DATE   GRADE

Haircoloring Portfolio...

Find examples of zonal haircoloring designs.

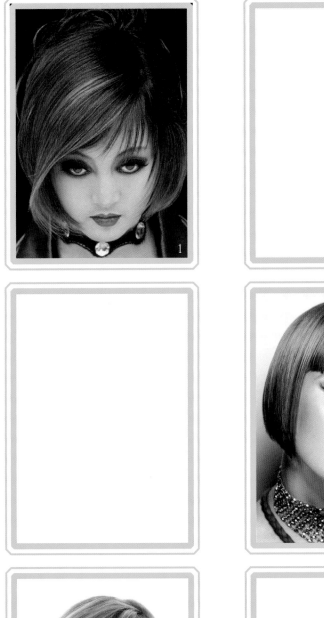

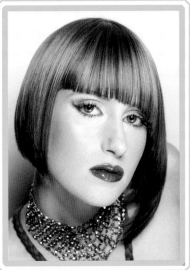

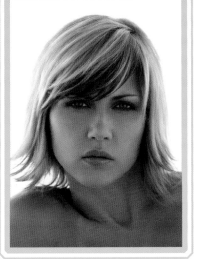

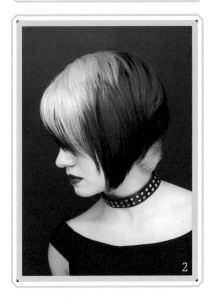

STUDENT'S NAME

DATE

GRADE

Haircoloring Portfolio ...

Find examples of fun colors.

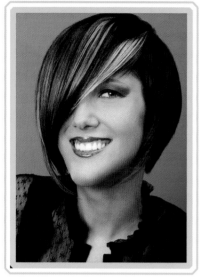

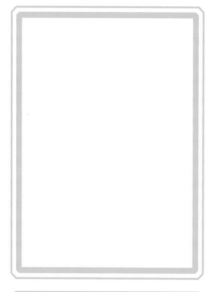

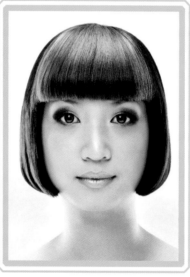

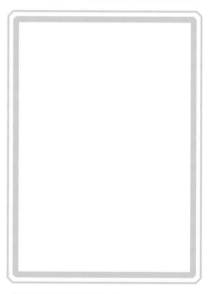

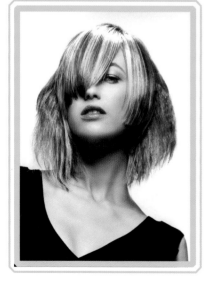

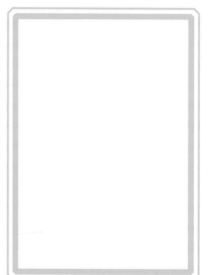

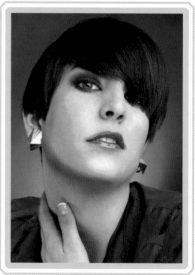

STUDENT'S NAME

DATE

GRADE

Haircoloring Portfolio...

Find examples of men's haircoloring.

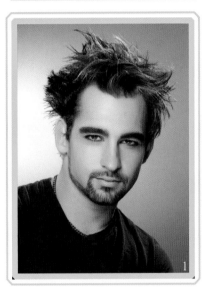

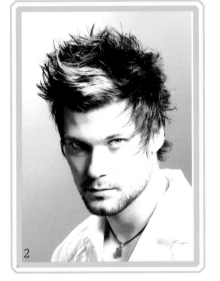

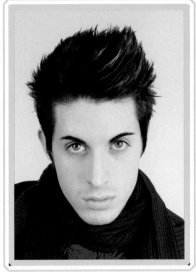

STUDENT'S NAME   DATE   GRADE

*Find examples of high
fashion haircolors.*

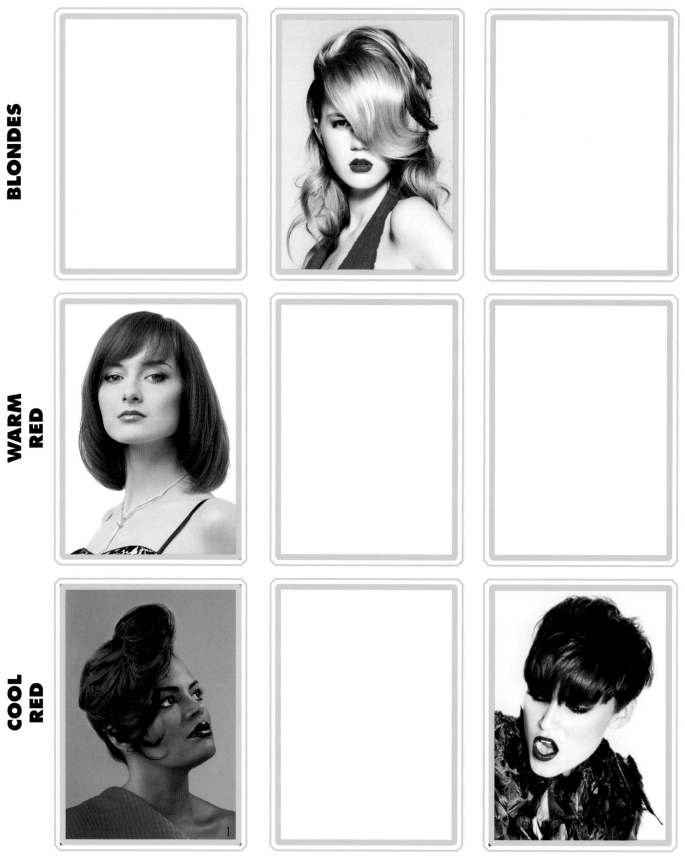

BLONDES

WARM RED

COOL RED

STUDENT'S NAME

DATE

GRADE

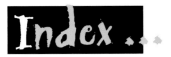

Index...

9 steps of haircoloring. *see* nine steps of haircoloring
10 steps of color separation, 181
10 volumes of hydrogen peroxide (H2O2), 52, 84, 179, 200
20 volumes of hydrogen peroxide (H2O2), 52, 84, 179, 200
30 volumes of hydrogen peroxide (H2O2), 52, 84, 179, 200
40 volumes of hydrogen peroxide (H2O2), 52, 84, 179, 200

A

acid pH, 86, 87, 89, 93
acquired canities, 119
action of hair lightener, 134, 139
action of haircolor, 129–133, 138
activator, 82
activities. *see* Lab Projects; student activities
African heritage, 159
afternoon light, 101
air purification system, 33
albinism, 119
alkaline pH, 86, 87, 89, 93
alkalizing agents, 82, 173
alkanolamines, 82, 85
allergies and allergic reactions
    defined, 16, 152
    latex, 28
    predisposition test, 152, 153, 204–205
    quick reference guide, 194
alpha helix coils, 115
American Board of Certified Hair Colorist, 10
amino acids, 77, 114, 115
aminomethyl propanol (AMP), 82
ammonia (NH3)
    action of haircolor, 133
    defined, 82
    haircolor chemistry, 82, 83
    pH, 89
AMP (aminomethyl propanol), 82
anagen, 127

ancestry, 158–159
aniline derivative. *see also* permanent haircolor
    defined, 92
    eyelashes and eyebrows, 153
    haircolor chemistry, 81, 133
    predisposition test, 152
    quick reference guide, 139
appearance, 147
applicator bottles, 36, 58
apron, 28
arrector pili, 112, 113
art of dimensional haircoloring, 229–258
    base dimensional color (star pattern), 248–249, 257
    flash color, 282–283
    foil pattern guide, 250–257
    free hand painting, 230–231
    highlighting
        cap and hook, 232–233
        with foils (full), 238–239, 252
        with foils (partial), 236–237, 251
        using crisscross pattern, 240–241, 253
    lowlighting with foils, 234–235, 250
    mathematics, 186–189
    overlays of color, 284–285
    ribbons of color, 244–245, 255, 278–279
    sponge spots, 280–281
    tone-on-tone coloring, 242–243, 254
    zone coloring, 246–247, 256, 278–279
    zones with ribbons of color, 278–279
art of haircoloring, 203–228
    color correction (tint black) lab, 224–225
    double process (lightener with toner), 222–223
    five-minute haircoloring lab, 226–227

gray coverage retouch, 220–221
permanent haircolor
    going darker, 212–213
    going lighter, 216–217
    going lighter retouch/refresh, 218–219
    retouch, 214–215
    predisposition test, 204–205
    semi-permanent haircolor, 210–211
    temporary haircolor, 208–209
ash family, 156–157, 165, 170, 196
Asian heritage, 159
atoms, 16, 76

B

baliage, 188, 231. *see also* free hand painting
base dimensional color (star pattern), 248–249, 257
base haircolor. *see* natural haircolor
base shape patterns, 189
beige series, 156–157, 166, 197
Big Bang theory, 62
biological powers, 95–140
    action of hair lightener, 134, 139
    action of haircolor, 129–133, 138
    color and emotion, 106
    color blindness, 99
    color therapy, 107
    hair, 110–113
        art with, 135
        composition, 114–115
        density, 122–123
        elasticity, 126
        growth of, 127–128
        porosity, 124–125
        texture, 120–121
    lighting types, 102–105
    natural haircolor, 116–119, 122, 137
    natural light, 100–101
    quick reference guide, 136–139
    review, 140
    student activities, 268
    surrounding color, 108–109

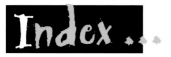

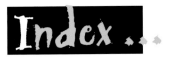
Index

concentrates, 51
conditioner filler, 51
conditioning, 190
congenital canities, 119
consultation, 144–150, 194, 214, 216, 218, 224, 226
continuing education, 10
cool colors, 68, 70, 74–75, 90, 155
cortex layer
   defined, 111, 137
   deposit, 17
   gray hair, 18
   melanin, 18
   structure, 115
cortical fibers, 115
cost efficient lighting, 104
cotton, 32
counterbalance guideline, 176
cream, protective, 32
cream hydrogen peroxide, 53
cream lighteners, 83
crisscross pattern highlighting, 240–241, 253
curly hair, 121
cuticle layer
   action of haircolor, 130, 131
   defined, 111, 137
   deposit, 17
   porosity, 21, 124
   structure, 115
cuticle scales, 115, 124

D

dawn, 100
daylight, 101, 102, 136
decapping, 17
decolorizing. *see also* lighteners and lightening
   chart of, 275
   chemistry, 83
   defined, 17
   stages of, 180–181
   student activities, 273–274
   with toner, 190
demarcation, line of, 19, 20, 79, 91
demi-permanent haircolor

action of haircolor, 129, 132, 138
   gray hair, 169
   haircoloring tools, 49
   oxidation and, 80
   pH, 89
   quick reference guide, 92
Democritus, 63
density, 122–123, 187
deposit, 17, 173
deposit-only color, 48, 234–235
dermal papilla, 112, 113
desired haircolor level, 164–167, 196–197
deuteranopia vision, 99
developer, 17
development/processing strand test, 206–207
diameter. *see* texture
dichromatism, 99
diffuse, 83
dilution, 178
dimensional haircoloring, 229–258
   base dimensional color (star pattern), 248–249, 257
   flash color, 282–283
   foil pattern guide, 250–257
   free hand painting, 230–231
   highlighting
      cap and hook, 232–233
      with foils (full), 238–239, 252
      with foils (partial), 236–237, 251
      using crisscross pattern, 240–241, 253
   lowlighting with foils, 234–235, 250
   mathematics, 186–189
   overlays of color, 284–285
   ribbons of color, 244–245, 255, 278–279
   sponge spots, 280–281
   tone-on-tone coloring, 242–243, 254
   zone coloring, 246–247, 256, 278–279

   zones with ribbons of color, 278–279
diode, 105
direct dye molecules, 78
disposable towels, 30
double process, 17, 190, 222–223
drabbers, 51
dramatic finish, 147, 188
draping, for haircoloring, 31
dry disinfection system, 33
dry hydrogen peroxide, 53
dusk, 101
dust masks, 33
dye intermediates, 133

E

early afternoon light, 101
early morning light, 100
Einstein, Albert, 63, 64
elasticity, 125, 126, 137
electrons, 76
element, 77
emotion, color and, 106
energy, light as, 64
Energy Independence and Security Act of 2007, 103
environment, salon
   client/guest record card, 145, 150, 193, 201, 276
   colors in, 108
   home-care use products, 86, 134, 193, 277
   lighting types, 96–98, 136
   retail display unit, 130
ethics, 145
eumelanin, 116, 117, 137, 160, 161
European heritage, 159
evaluation. *see also* review; student activities
   base dimensional color (star pattern), 248–249
   color correction (tint black), 224–225
   double process (lightener with toner), 222–223

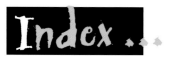

Index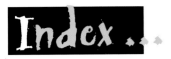

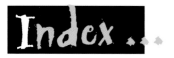

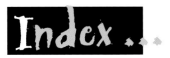

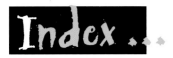

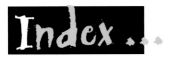

CLiC Classmates Sign In ...

School ————————————————— Class of —————————————————

Thank you for joining our professional team
of great haircolorists!